T0325354

Interpretation Basics of Cone Beam Computed Tomography

Interpretation Basics of Cone Beam Computed Tomography

Second Edition

Edited by

Shawneen M. Gonzalez
DDS, MS, Diplomate,
American Board of Oral and
Maxillofacial Radiology with
invited Contribution from
Gayle Tieszen Reardon

WILEY Blackwell

Registered Office
John Wiley & Sons, Inc., 111 River Street, Hoboken, NJ 07030, USA

Editorial Office
111 River Street, Hoboken, NJ 07030, USA

For details of our global editorial offices, customer services, and more information about Wiley products visit us at www.wiley.com.

Wiley also publishes its books in a variety of electronic formats and by print-on-demand. Some content that appears in standard print versions of this book may not be available in other formats.

Limit of Liability/Disclaimer of Warranty
The contents of this work are intended to further general scientific research, understanding, and discussion only and are not intended and should not be relied upon as recommending or promoting scientific method, diagnosis, or treatment by physicians for any particular patient. In view of ongoing research, equipment modifications, changes in governmental regulations, and the constant flow of information relating to the use of medicines, equipment, and devices, the reader is urged to review and evaluate the information provided in the package insert or instructions for each medicine, equipment, or device for, among other things, any changes in the instructions or indication of usage and for added warnings and precautions. While the publisher and authors have used their best efforts in preparing this work, they make no representations or warranties with respect to the accuracy or completeness of the contents of this work and specifically disclaim all warranties, including without limitation any implied warranties of merchantability or fitness for a particular purpose. No warranty may be created or extended by sales representatives, written sales materials or promotional statements for this work. The fact that an organization, website, or product is referred to in this work as a citation and/or potential source of further information does not mean that the publisher and authors endorse the information or services the organization, website, or product may provide or recommendations it may make. This work is sold with the understanding that the publisher is not engaged in rendering professional services. The advice and strategies contained herein may not be suitable for your situation. You should consult with a specialist where appropriate. Further, readers should be aware that websites listed in this work may have changed or disappeared between when this work was written and when it is read. Neither the publisher nor authors shall be liable for any loss of profit or any other commercial damages, including but not limited to special, incidental, consequential, or other damages.

Library of Congress Cataloging-in-Publication Data

Names: Gonzalez, Shawneen, author, editor.
Title: Interpretation basics of cone beam computed tomography / edited by
    Shawneen M. Gonzalez.
Description: Second edition. | Hoboken, NJ : Wiley-Blackwell 2021. |
    Includes bibliographical references and index.
Identifiers: LCCN 2021028942 (print) | LCCN 2021028943 (ebook) | ISBN
    9781119685845 (hardback) | ISBN 9781119685852 (adobe pdf) | ISBN
    9781119685876 (epub)
Subjects: MESH: Cone-Beam Computed Tomography. | Radiography,
    Dental–methods. | Craniofacial Abnormalities–diagnosis. | Facial Bones
Classification: LCC RC78.7.T6 (print) | LCC RC78.7.T6 (ebook) | NLM WN
    230 | DDC 616.07/5722–dc23
LC record available at https://lccn.loc.gov/2021028942
LC ebook record available at https://lccn.loc.gov/2021028943

Cover Design: Wiley
Cover Image: © Shawneen M. Gonzalez

Set in 10/12pt Sabon by Straive, Pondicherry, India

Printed in Singapore
M106570_260721

Contents

Preface to the Second Edition

It is the goal of this book to help practitioners and students gain a better understanding of anatomy and common disease processes that frequently present on cone beam computed tomography (CBCT) scans. This book seeks to fill the gap in the current literature where little is presented on common radiographic appearances on CBCT. In addition to this book, there are sample cases with videos online at www.wiley.com/go/gonzalez/interpretation, where you can practice working your way through regions and entire scans using the knowledge you acquire in this book.

The beginning of the book covers general information about different CBCT unit parameters and recommended uses from specialty organizations. The third chapter covers legal considerations of owning a cone beam CT, referring patients for a cone beam CT scan, and/or interpreting cone beam CT scans in the United States. This information is lacking in the current literature and is something many professionals should be aware of before purchasing or using a cone beam CT unit.

Each book chapter from the fourth chapter on is an anatomical region covering the topics of anatomy, common anatomic variants/developmental anomalies, pathosis, and other findings. The first regions presented are the paranasal sinuses and mastoid air cells and nasal cavity and airway, which are intimately involved with each other. The anatomy section covers pertinent anatomy to evaluate when interpreting or reviewing a scan. The next section covers common anatomic variants with various images showing how they appear on axial, coronal, and sagittal views. The last section covers commonly seen disease processes, such as sinusitis, that should be noted on a written radiology interpretation.

Chapter 6 is on the cranial skull base and orbits. There are many anatomical landmarks in the cranial skull base such as canals, foramina, air cells, and more, making this a difficult region to interpret. Key anatomy is shown on various views (axial, coronal, and sagittal) to aid CBCT users in orienting themselves on the scan.

All soft-tissue findings are moved into one chapter. There is no anatomy as CBCT is a hard-tissue imaging modality. All findings are listed as pathosis or other findings and appear as calcifications in the soft tissues.

The region of the cervical spine covers anatomy to disease processes such as degenerative joint disease. Degenerative joint disease is progressive with multiple appearances based on the degree of bony damage. This chapter has many example images of degenerative joint disease at various points in the disease process.

The last region covered is the temporomandibular joints, which is very thorough thanks to the contributions of Gayle Reardon, who has studied and continues to study this region in depth. The temporomandibular joints have a unique set of disease processes and developmental appearances beyond arthritic changes. This chapter covers entities CBCT users should be aware of even if they are not seen in daily practice.

The appendix shows example written reports of CBCT scans to view and consider when writing radiology interpretations.

Acknowledgments

I'd like to thank Gayle Reardon for her contributions to this book and sharing her knowledge of the paranasal sinuses, nasal cavity and airway, temporomandibular joints, and implants. Thanks to the staff at Wiley for guidance and support in the creation of this book. Last, a giant thanks to my family (Max, Max, and Rugen) for their love, support, and encouragement throughout this entire process. I would not have been able to complete this without them.

About the Companion Website

Do not forget to visit the companion website for this book:

www.wiley.com/go/gonzalez/interpretation

▪ Sample cases with videos

Scan this QR code to visit the companion website:

Introduction to Cone Beam Computed Tomography

Shawneen M. Gonzalez

Introduction

This chapter covers basics of cone beam computed tomography including comparison to traditional computed tomography, artifacts frequently seen, and views created with a cone beam computed tomography dataset.

Conventional Computed Tomography

General Information

Computed tomography (CT) is credited to Godfrey Hounsfield, who in 1967 wrote about the technology and then created a unit in 1972. He was awarded the Nobel Prize in Physiology/Medicine in 1979. Conventional CT units are both hard-tissue and soft-tissue imaging modalities. The first CT, first generation, had a scan time of 10+ minutes depending on how much of the body was being imaged. The processing time would take 2½ hours or longer. All first-generation CT units were only a single slice. This means that one fan of radiation exposed the patient and would have to circle around the patient several times to cover the area of concern. Current CT units are fifth generation, or helical/spiral. The scan times have gone down to 20–60 seconds with a processing time of 2–20 minutes. The number of slices available is up to 64, 128, 256, and 512+. The more slices available makes it possible to scan more of the patient in one circle, hence the shorter scan times. Conventional CT units work with the patient lying down on a table while being scanned. The table moves in and out of the bore to cover the area of concern. Once all the data are received,

Interpretation Basics of Cone Beam Computed Tomography, Second Edition.
Edited by Shawneen M. Gonzalez.
© 2021 John Wiley & Sons, Inc. Published 2021 by John Wiley & Sons, Inc.
Companion website: www.wiley.com/go/gonzalez/interpretation

they are compiled to create a dataset. This dataset can be manipulated to look at the information in many different angles.

Cone Beam Computed Tomography

General Information

Cone beam computed tomography (CBCT) was developed in Italy in 1997. The first unit created was the NewTom. The NewTom was similar to conventional CT in having the patient lying down with an open bore where the radiation exposes the patient. Instead of a fan of radiation (used in conventional CT units), a cone of radiation is used to expose the patient, hence the name cone beam computed tomography. As new CBCT units were created, companies started using seated or standing options. With continued updates to the units, the sizes have become smaller, with many needing only as much space as a pantomograph machine.

Conventional CT versus Cone Beam CT

Voxels

Voxels are 3D data blocks representing a specific x-ray absorption. CBCT units capture isotropic voxels. An isotropic voxel is equal in all three dimensions (x, y, and z planes), producing higher-resolution images compared to conventional CT units. Conventional CT unit voxels are non-isotropic with two sides equal, but the third side (z-plane) different. The voxel sizes currently available in CBCT units range from 0.076 mm to 0.6 mm. The voxel sizes currently available in conventional CT units range from 1.25 mm to 5.0 mm. Resolution of the final image is determined by the unit's voxel size. The smaller the voxel size the higher the resolution.

Field of View

Field of view (FOV) is the area of the patient captured. CBCT units vary in FOV options, with some units having a fixed FOV and some having variable FOVs. The ranges of FOVs are from 5 cm × 3.8 cm, commonly referred to as a small/quadrant FOV, to 23 cm × 26 cm, commonly referred to as a large FOV (Figures 1.1–1.6).

Radiation Doses

Radiation doses with CBCT units are as varied as the FOV options. CBCT units have approximate radiation dose ranges of 5 microSieverts to 1073 microSieverts. Conventional CT units have much higher radiation doses due to their soft tissue capabilities, with doses of 1200 microSieverts and higher per each scan, depending on the selected scan field.

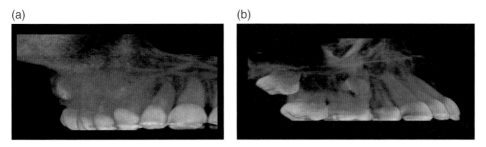

Figure 1.1. (a) 3D rendering of a small FOV of 5 cm × 8 cm from an anteroposterior (AP) view. (b) 3D rendering of a small FOV of 5 cm × 8 cm from a lateral view.

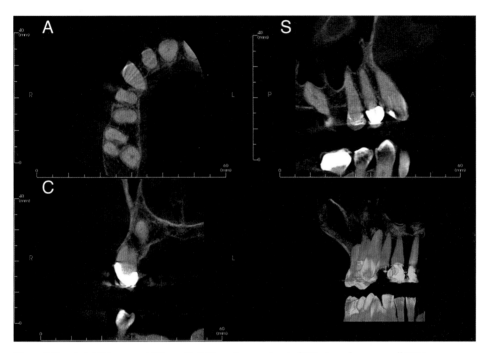

Figure 1.2. Axial (A), coronal (C), sagittal (S), and reconstructed 3D views from a small FOV.

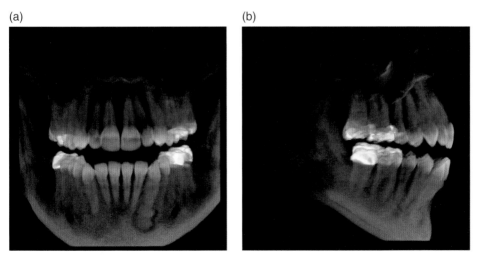

Figure 1.3. (a) 3D rendering of a medium FOV of 8 cm × 8 cm from an anteroposterior (AP) view. (b) 3D rendering of a medium FOV of 8 cm × 8 cm from a lateral view.

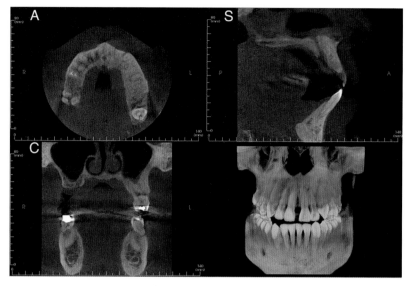

Figure 1.4.   Axial (A), coronal (C), sagittal (S), and reconstructed 3D views from medium FOV.

(a)   (b)

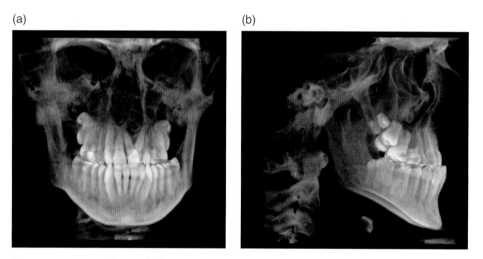

Figure 1.5.   (a) 3D rendering of a large FOV of 16 cm × 16 cm from an anteroposterior (AP) view. (b) 3D rendering of a large FOV of 16 cm × 16 cm from a lateral view.

Viewing CBCT Data

Multiplanar Reformation

Multiplanar reformation, or MPR, is a view of three different directional 2D images (axial, coronal, and sagittal planes) (Figure 1.7). Within this view, the images may be manipulated in the thickness of data, and direction of viewing can be altered. Reconstructed pantomographs and lateral cephalometric skulls (Figures 1.8 and 1.9) are possible without distortion from standard 2D radiography. The dataset may also be manipulated to create cross-sectional (orthogonal) views of the jaws and condyles (Figures 1.10 and 1.11).

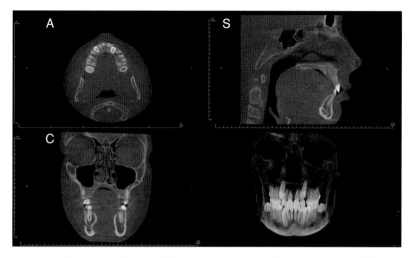

Figure 1.6.   Axial (A), coronal (C), sagittal (S), and reconstructed 3D views from large FOV.

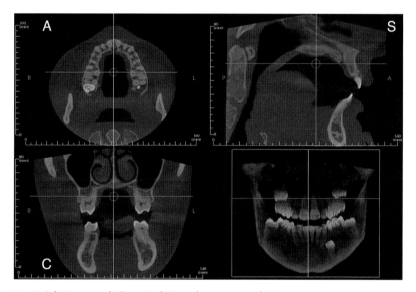

Figure 1.7.   Axial (A), coronal (C), sagittal (S), and reconstructed 3D views.

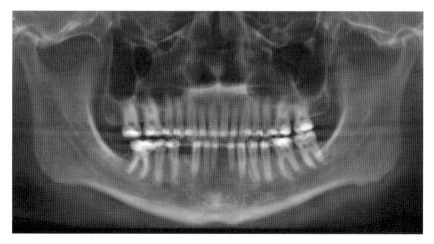

Figure 1.8.   Reconstructed pantomograph from a CBCT scan.

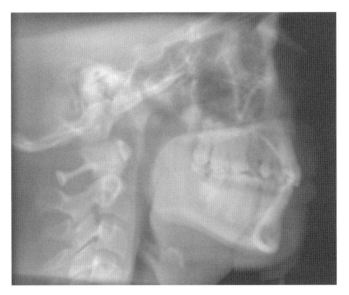

Figure 1.9.   Reconstructed lateral cephalometric skull.

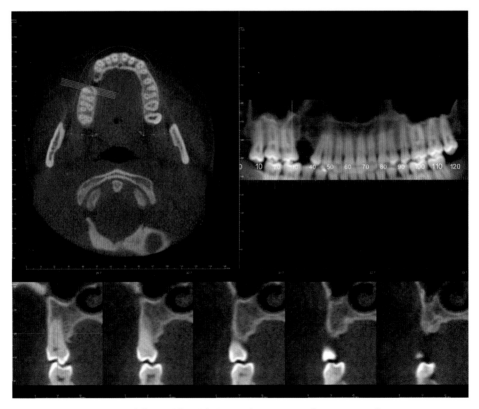

Figure 1.10.   Cross-sectional slices with axial view and reconstructed pantomograph.

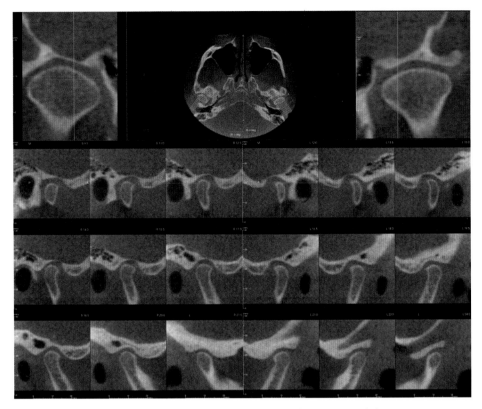

Figure 1.11. Temporomandibular joint view with rotated sagittal cross-sectional slices.

3D Rendering

The most common form of 3D rendering offered in CBCT software is indirect volume rendering, which determines the grays of the voxels to create a 3D image (Figure 1.12). Another form of 3D rendering is referred to as direct volume rendering, where the highest attenuation value for each voxel is used creating a maximum intensity projection (MIP) (Figure 1.13).

Artifacts

Streak Artifacts/Undersampling

Streak artifacts occur when an object with high density (such as metallic restorations) creates areas of undersampling where no viable information is recorded. These present as white streaks (Figure 1.14) radiating from the high-density object. Beam hardening artifact is caused when low energy x-rays are absorbed by high-density objects creating an increase in x-ray beam energy, which "hardens" the beam. This results as increased density (black) lines radiating from the high-density object (Figure 1.14). Care should be taken not to interpret anything in the streak artifacts

(a)   (b)

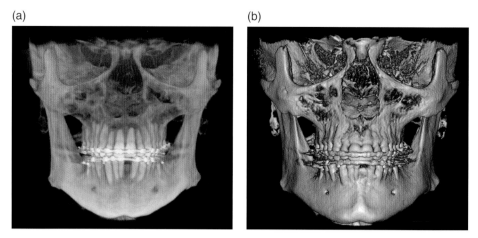

Figure 1.12.   (a) 3D rendered view with teeth setting. (b) 3D rendered view with bone setting.

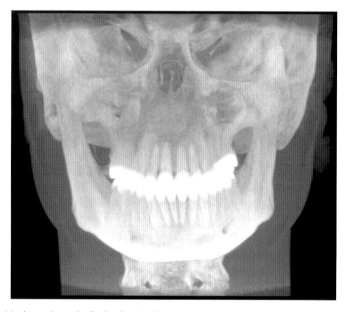

Figure 1.13.   Maximum Intensity Projection (MIP) view.

and beam hardening. Aliasing is another form of undersampling, when too few images are acquired and appear as small lines throughout a scan (Figure 1.15).

Motion Artifacts

Motion artifacts occur due to either normal pathophysiological movement or when the patient moves during a scan. This presents as double bony borders to ill-defined bony borders (Figures 1.16 and 1.17). This can be minimized by restraining the patient's head and using as short a scan time as possible.

(a)   (b)

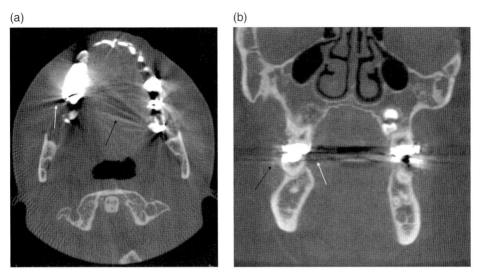

Figure 1.14. (a) Axial view showing streak artifact (black arrow) and beam hardening (white arrow) due to metallic restorations. (b) Coronal view showing streak artifact (black arrow) and beam hardening (white arrow) due to metallic restorations.

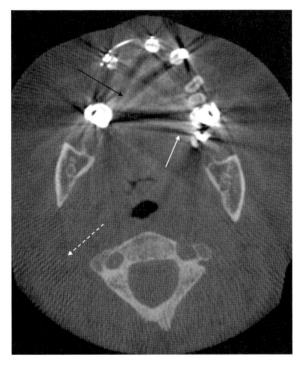

Figure 1.15. Axial view with metallic streak artifact (black arrow), beam hardening (white arrow), and aliasing of scan as linear radiolucent lines (white dotted arrow) throughout the entire image.

Ring Artifacts

Ring artifacts present as white or black circular artifacts. They typically indicate poor calibrations and imperfections in the scanner detection (Figure 1.18).

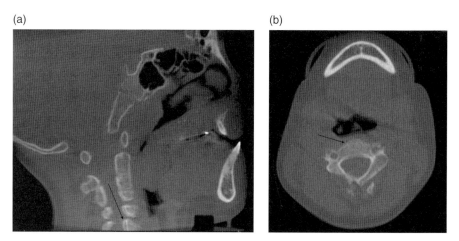

Figure 1.16. (a) Sagittal view showing motion artifact of the cervical vertebrae (black arrow). (b) Axial view showing motion artifact of the cervical vertebrae (black arrow).

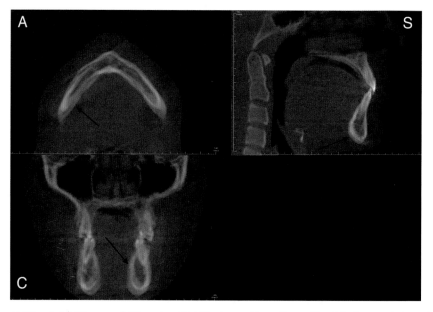

Figure 1.17. Axial (A), coronal (C), and sagittal (S) views with motion artifact (black arrows) throughout the jaws.

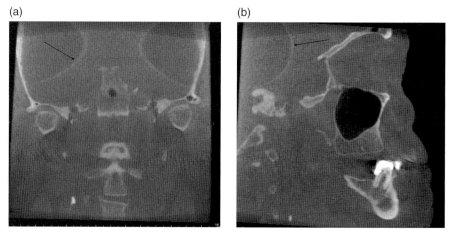

Figure 1.18. (a) Coronal view showing white ring artifacts (black arrow). (b) Sagittal view showing white ring artifacts (black arrow).

References

Conventional Computed Tomography and Cone Beam Computed Tomography

Dalrymple, N. C., Prasad, S. R., El-Merhi, F. M., et al. (2007). Price of isotropy in multidetector CT. *RadioGraphics*, **27**, 49–62.

Hounsfield, G. (1973). Computerized transverse axial scanning (tomography). 1. Description of the system. *Br J Radiol*, **46**, 1016–22.

Mallaya, S., and Lam, E. (Ed.). (2019). *White and Pharaoh's Oral Radiology: Principles and Interpretation*. Mosby.

Miles, D. E. (2008). *Color Atlas of Cone Beam Volumetric Imaging for Dental Applications*. Quintessence.

Popat, H., Drage, N., Durning, P. (2008). Mid-line clefts of the cervical vertebrae— an incidental finding arising from cone beam computed tomography of the dental patient. *Br Dental J*, **204**, 303–6.

Viewing CBCT Data

Cody, D. D. (2002). AAPM/RSNA physics tutorial for residents: topics in CT. *Image processing in CT. Radiographics*, **22**, 1255–68.

Mallaya, S., and Lam, E. (Ed.). (2019). *White and Pharaoh's Oral Radiology: Principles and Interpretation*. Mosby.

Artifacts

Mallaya, S., and Lam, E. (Ed.). (2019). *White and Pharaoh's Oral Radiology: Principles and Interpretation*. Mosby.

Pauwels, R., Araki, K., Siewerdsen, J. H., et. al. (2015). Technical aspects of dental CBCT: state of the art. *Dentomaxillofac Radiol*, **44**, 20140224.

Popilock, R., Sandrasagaren, K., Harris, L., et al. (2008). CT artifact recognition for the nuclear technologist. *J Nucl Med Technol*, **36**, 79–81.

Zoller, J. E., and Nuegebauer, J. (2008). *Cone-Beam Volumetric Imaging in Dental, Oral, and Maxillofacial Medicine*. Quintessence, Germany.

Cone Beam Computed Tomography Recommendations

2

Shawneen M. Gonzalez

Introduction

This chapter covers cone beam computed tomography recommendations and guidelines regarding use and imaging. The areas covered include recommendations from American endodontics, orthodontics, and periodontics specialty organizations along with sample cases.

Endodontics

The American Association of Endodontics (AAE) and the American Academy of Oral and Maxillofacial Radiology (AAOMR) have come out with two position papers regarding cone beam computed tomography (CBCT) use in endodontics.

2010 Position Paper

There were two main imaging goals from the 2010 paper – field of view (FOV) and resolution/voxel size. A small/limited FOV and a resolution/voxel size of 0.2 mm or smaller is recommended. This combination allows better visualization for small changes to the periodontal ligament space, bone, and teeth. When using CBCT, it should not be used for routine use and should be based on a patient's history and clinical examination. Before capturing a CBCT scan, it is important to receive patient consent and explain the risks and benefits of the imaging modality. Last, the entire CBCT volume must be interpreted.

Interpretation Basics of Cone Beam Computed Tomography, Second Edition.
Edited by Shawneen M. Gonzalez.
© 2021 John Wiley & Sons, Inc. Published 2021 by John Wiley & Sons, Inc.
Companion website: www.wiley.com/go/gonzalez/interpretation

2015/2016 Update

The updated position paper gives 14 case examples and whether a limited FOV CBCT or intraoral 2D imaging is recommended. They are separated into different categories: diagnosis, initial treatment, nonsurgical treatment, surgical retreatment, special conditions, and outcome assessment.

Diagnosis

1 = Intraoral radiographs should be considered for the evaluation of endodontic patients.

2 = Limited FOV CBCT should be considered when there are nonspecific clinical signs or symptoms with an untreated or previously endodontically treated tooth.

CBCT imaging has increased sensitivity in the detection of periapical pathosis (Figure 2.1) compared to intraoral radiographs. In the presence of clinical signs with the absence of intraoral radiographic findings, a CBCT may be recommended to rule out or rule in possible periapical pathosis. It is important to thoroughly check all of the teeth on a scan because early periapical pathosis has been noted on CBCT prior to detection on intraoral radiographs. Sagittal and cross-sectional views are the recommended views for detecting periapical pathosis.

Initial Treatment

3 = Limited FOV CBCT should be considered when evaluating teeth with potential extra canals or complex morphology (excludes maxillary incisors) (Figure 2.2).

4 = Limited FOV CBCT should be considered to identify and localize calcified canals.

5 = Intraoral radiographs should be considered for immediate postoperative evaluation.

Nonsurgical Treatment

6 = Limited FOV CBCT should be considered if the clinical exam and intraoral radiographs are inconclusive for detecting a vertical root fracture.

Vertical root fractures are difficult to diagnose on intraoral radiographs with localized bone changes visualized first (Figure 2.3). The bone changes typically

(a)   (b)

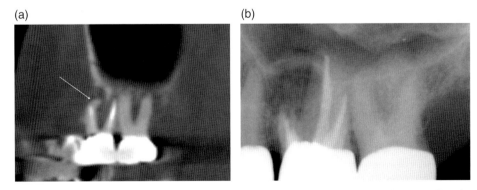

Figure 2.1.   (a) Sagittal view showing a distal dilaceration of the mesio-buccal root of the maxillary first molar with a short endodontic filling and rarefying osteitis (white arrow). (b) Periapical radiograph showing a resulting apicoectomy after the findings on the CBCT scan.

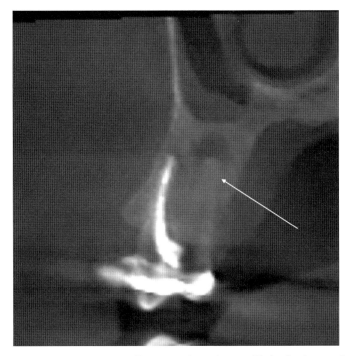

Figure 2.2. Coronal view showing a maxillary premolar with an unfilled palatal root (white arrow) and apical rarefying osteitis.

(a)   (b)

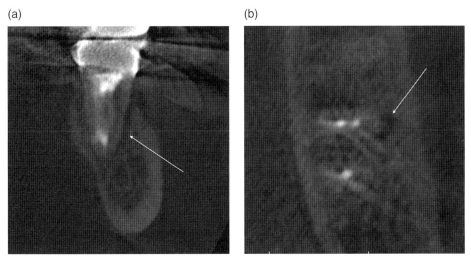

Figure 2.3. (a) Coronal view showing localized vertical bone loss (white arrow) along the facial root surface of a mandible molar. (b) Axial view showing localized bone loss (white arrow) along the facial root surface of a mandible molar.

present with J-shaped bone loss around the root with the fracture. CBCT imaging has increased sensitivity in detecting vertical and horizontal root fractures (Figures 2.4 and 2.5). Coronal, sagittal, and cross-sectional views are the recommended views for detecting vertical root fractures. One concern when evaluating for fractures is teeth that have been endodontically treated, as the filling material causes artifacts that obscure small fractures and create pseudo-fracture lines (Figure 2.6).

(a)

(b)

(c)

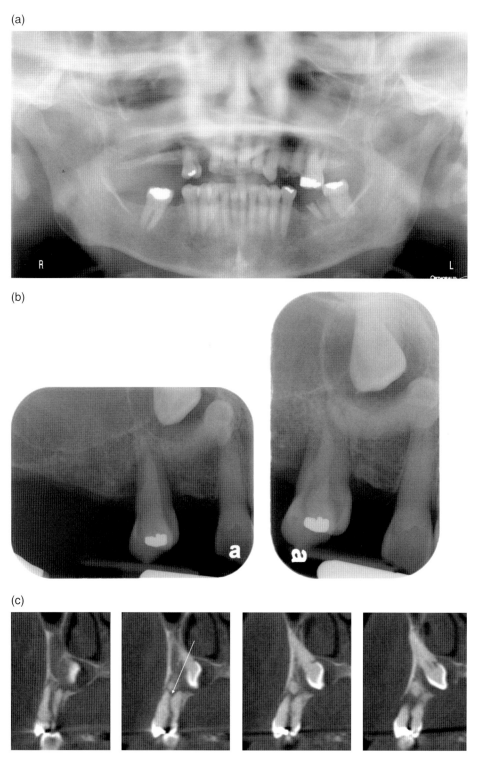

Figure 2.4.   (a) Pantomograph showing impacted maxillary right canine. (b) Periapical radiographs showing impacted maxillary right first premolar and canine with a dentigerous cyst. (c) Cross-sectional slices showing a vertical root fracture on the maxillary right second premolar (white arrow) and dentigerous cyst associated with impacted canine.

(a)

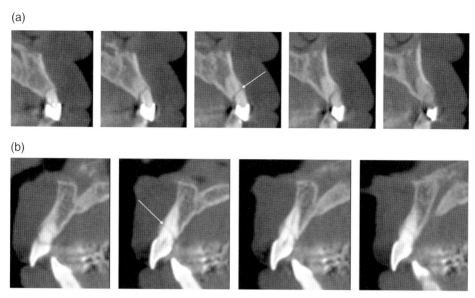

(b)

Figure 2.5. (a) Cross-sectional slices showing a horizontal root fracture (white arrow). (b) Cross-sectional slices showing a horizontal root fracture (white arrow).

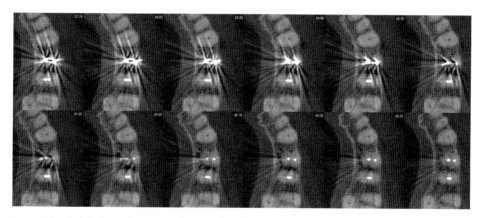

Figure 2.6. Axial views showing artifact streaking from an endodontically treated tooth obscuring the root when evaluating for root fractures.

The smallest root fracture that can be visualized on a CBCT scan is determined by the resolution/voxel size used. This is due to the Nyquist Theorem, which samples digitized information at 2 times the highest frequency. On a CBCT scan, this translates to the smallest root fracture visualized is twice the resolution/voxel size used. For example, if a resolution/voxel size of 0.2 mm is used, the smallest root fracture visible would be 0.4 mm.

7 = Limited FOV CBCT should be considered when evaluating nonhealing previous endodontic treatment.

8 = Limited FOV CBCT should be considered for nonsurgical retreatment.

Surgical Retreatment

9 = Limited FOV CBCT should be considered for presurgical treatment planning.

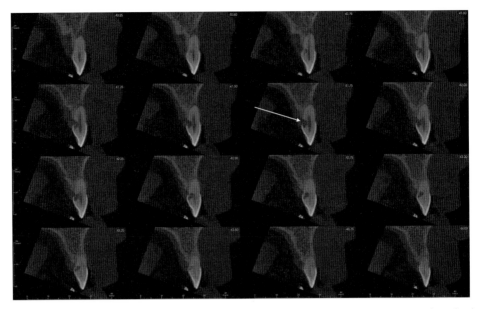

Figure 2.7.   Sagittal views showing the extent of invasive cervical resorption (white arrow) on the palatal root surface of a maxillary incisor.

Special Conditions

10 = Limited FOV CBCT should be considered for implant treatment planning and placement.

11 = Limited FOV CBCT should be considered for diagnosis and management after trauma.

12 = Limited FOV CBCT should be considered for localizing resorption (Figures 2.7 and 2.8).

Outcome Assessment

13 = Intraoral radiographs should be considered when evaluating healing post-non-surgical or surgical endodontic treatment if no clinical signs or symptoms are present.

HOWEVER
14 = Limited FOV CBCT should be considered if it was used pretreatment to re-evaluate the tooth endodontically treated (Figure 2.9).

Orthodontics

The AAOMR published a paper in 2013 with recommendations regarding CBCT use in orthodontics. There are four main guidelines given.

1 = Image appropriately according to the patient's clinical condition.
Imaging should be based on a patient's history, clinical examination, and presence of clinical findings where CBCT benefits outweigh risks. Avoid using a CBCT only for lateral cephalometric and panoramic views or when information can be obtained

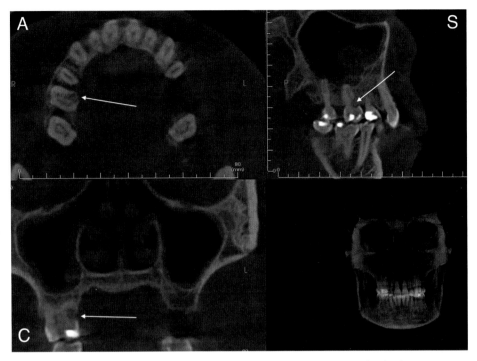

Figure 2.8.   Axial (A), coronal (C) and sagittal (S) views showing the extent of palatal root resorption (white arrow) of the maxillary right first molar.

with nonionizing methods such as virtual models. When using CBCT, a FOV that captures only the region of interest should be used.

2 = Assess the radiation dose risk.

Consider the relative radiation level when assessing imaging risk over the course of orthodontic treatment. Explain risks and benefits to patients prior to imaging and document in patients records.

3 = Minimize patient radiation exposure.

Take a CBCT with proper settings, a FOV that matches the region of interest, adult versus child setting, and appropriate voxel size. Use shielding when possible, but make sure that it is not captured in the FOV (Figure 2.10). If you have a CBCT unit in office, ensure the machine is continually calibrated.

4 = Maintain professional competency in performing and interpreting CBCT studies.

Practitioners should continually attend continuing education (CE) courses, staying informed of the latest CBCT information. Practitioners have a legal responsibility to comply with local laws regarding CBCT use and interpretation. Patients should be informed of CBCT limitations (not a soft-tissue imaging modality, artifacts, etc.).

Specific Orthodontic Uses

In 2015, Fisher recommended a list of case types for CBCT imaging in orthodontics.

1 = Impacted canines.

The most commonly impacted teeth are third molars and maxillary canines. CBCT imaging provides exact locations of impacted canines and the presence or

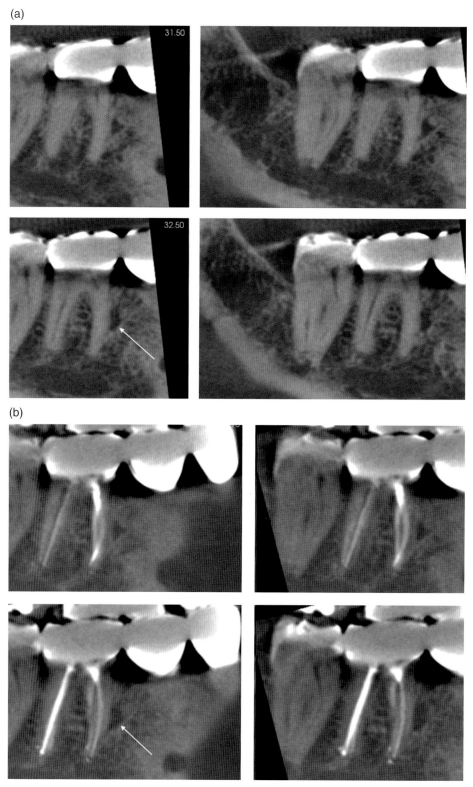

Figure 2.9. (a) Rotated sagittal views showing a bone defect (white arrow) on the mesial of a mandibular molar. (b) Rotated sagittal views showing a bone defect (white arrow) on the mesial of a mandibular molar captured 6 months after (a) suggestive of a prominent marrow space.

(a)

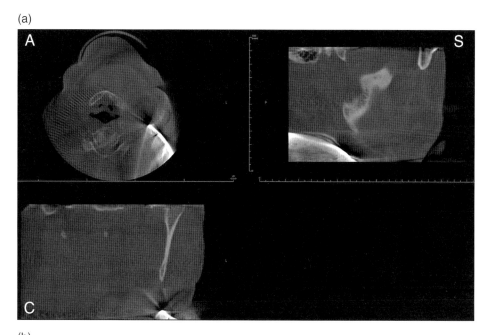

(b)

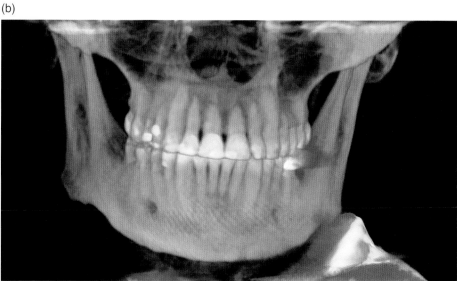

Figure 2.10.   (a) Axial (A), coronal (C), and sagittal (S) views showing a thyroid collar captured in the FOV. (b) 3D reconstruction showing a thyroid collar captured in the FOV.

absence of external root resorption of adjacent teeth (Figures 2.11 and 2.12). Cross-sectional views are recommended to determine exact facial-lingual width and effect on adjacent teeth. The FOV recommended is large enough to capture the tooth or teeth in question and surrounding bone and anatomical structures. The recommended voxel size is 0.3 mm to reduce the overall radiation exposure.

2 = Orthognavthic surgery.

   CBCT imaging has shown limited research that scans are reliable when determining the bony dimensions of a cleft palate (Figure 2.13). Cleft palate cases are recommended for CBCT imaging, as 2D radiographs cannot show facial-lingual

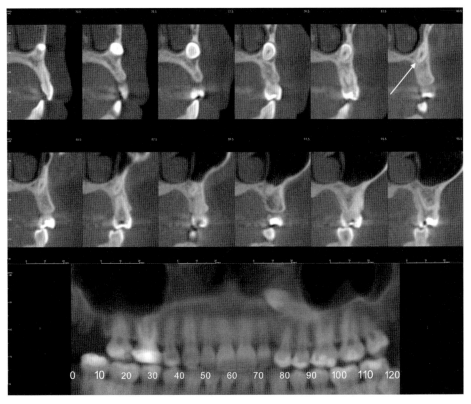

Figure 2.11. Reconstructed pantomograph and cross-sectional slices showing location of an impacted maxillary canine (white arrow).

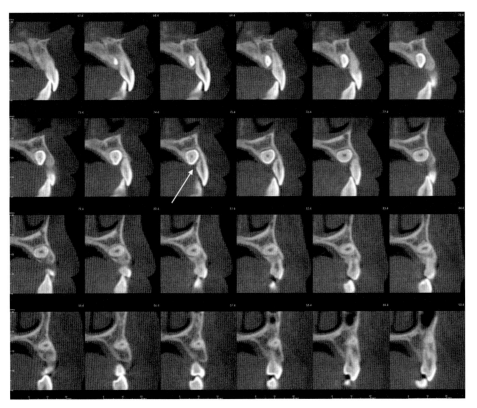

Figure 2.12. Cross-sectional slices of an impacted maxillary canine with external resorption on the lingual aspect of the lateral incisor (white arrow).

(a)　　　　　　　　　　　　　　　　　(b)

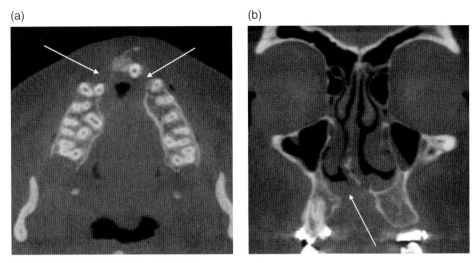

Figure 2.13. (a) Axial view showing a bilateral cleft palate (white arrows). (b) Coronal view showing a discontinuity of the floor of the right nasal cavity associated with a cleft palate (white arrow).

dimensions of a defect. This additional information is helpful to a surgeon especially prior to bone grafting and helpful to an orthodontist prior to movement of teeth near the defect. Axial views are recommended to determine the bone quantity surrounding roots of teeth adjacent to the cleft. The FOV recommended is large enough to see the entire cleft and portions of the nasal cavity for the surgeon to have all of the information necessary. The recommended voxel size is 0.3 mm or larger, so as to reduce the overall radiation exposure.

3 = Any patient needing anterior teeth moved in the sagittal plane.

4 = Temporary anchorage devices.

5 = Maxillary expansion.

6 = Permanent implant (see Chapter 11 for more information).

7 = Compromised airway.

8 = Temporomandibular joint disorder (TMD) (see Chapter 10 for more information).

9 = Supernumerary teeth (Figure 2.14).

10 = Pathology.

There are various bony lesions that present throughout the jaws (Figures 2.15 and 2.16). CBCT imaging provides additional information about the exact location and possible nature of a bony lesion prior to removal or biopsy. All views (axial, coronal, sagittal, and cross-sectional) are recommended to completely grasp the size, position, and nature of a lesion. The FOV recommended is one large enough to capture the area in question. The recommended voxel size is 0.3 mm to reduce the overall radiation exposure.

(a)

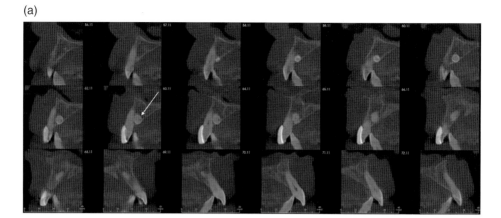

(b)

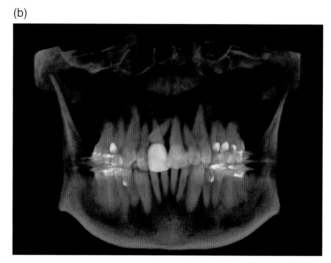

Figure 2.14.   (a) Cross-sectional slices showing a supernumerary tooth position (white arrow) in relation to the erupted maxillary incisors. (b) 3D reconstruction showing a supernumerary tooth horizontally positioned.

Periodontics

The American Academy of Periodontology (AAP) created a set of questions regarding CBCT use based on published research in 2017. They asked three main questions when reviewing CBCT research, covering goals, benefits, potential risks, and the bottom line.

Implants

"Should CBCT imaging replace two-dimensional (2D) radiographic analysis of regional anatomy in the surgical management of patients requiring dental implants?"

Goals

- Diagnosis and treatment outcome assessment.
- Implant treatment planning.
- Anatomic characterization.

Benefits

CBCT helped to identify incidental findings that may influence treatment including but not limited to anatomic variants, pathologies and fractures. CBCT supports minimally invasive therapy for dental implants and provides a method to educate patients.

Quantity of bone, alveolar ridge morphology, maxillary sinus location, and mandibular canal location are important information prior to placing an implant. Standard intraoral radiographs provide the height of bone available but do not show whether there are ridge defects or concavities (Figures 2.17 and 2.18). CBCT imaging provides information on these things to ensure implant placement within the bone and not surrounding soft tissues. Cross-sectional views are recommended to view the facial-lingual width and morphology of the alveolar ridge. The recommended voxel size is 0.3 mm to reduce the overall radiation exposure.

(a)

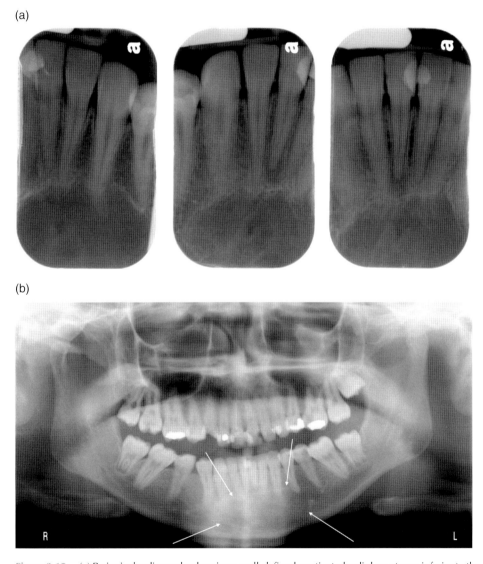

(b)

Figure 2.15. (a) Periapical radiographs showing a well-defined, corticated radiolucent area inferior to the apices of the mandibular incisors confirmed as an odontogenic myxoma histopathologically. (b) Pantomograph showing a well-defined radiolucent area in the anterior mandible (white arrows) confirmed as an odontogenic myxoma histopathologically.

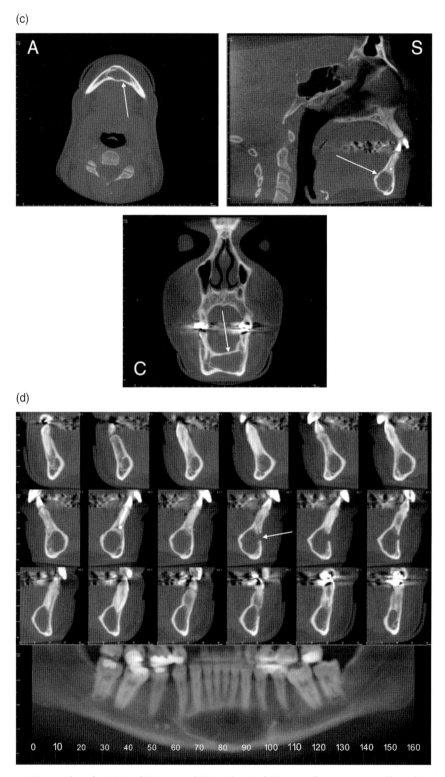

Figure 2.15. (*continued*)   (c) Axial (A), coronal (C), and sagittal (S) views showing extent of bone loss associated with the odontogenic myxoma (white arrows). (d) Reconstructed pantomograph and cross-sectional slices showing width of odontogenic myxoma. Bone discontinuity on the facial cortical plate from a prior incisional biopsy (white arrow).

Potential Risks

Long-term radiation hazards of effective dose accumulation are still unknown, so the practitioner should minimize exposure when possible.

Bottom Line

CBCT should be used as an adjunct to 2D imaging when the benefits outweigh the risks.

Tooth Movement

"Is CBCT imaging useful in determining risk to periodontal structures in patients requiring tooth movement?"

(a)

(b)

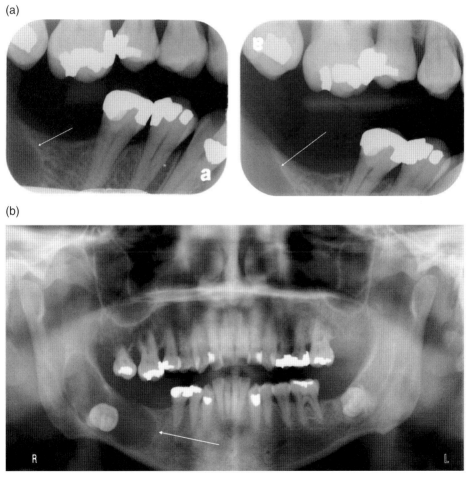

Figure 2.16.   (a) Bitewing radiographs showing bone loss (white arrow) in the mandible. (b) Pantomograph showing a well-defined, corticated, ovoid radiolucent area around an impacted mandibular right third molar (white arrow) consistent with a dentigerous cyst.

(c)

(d)

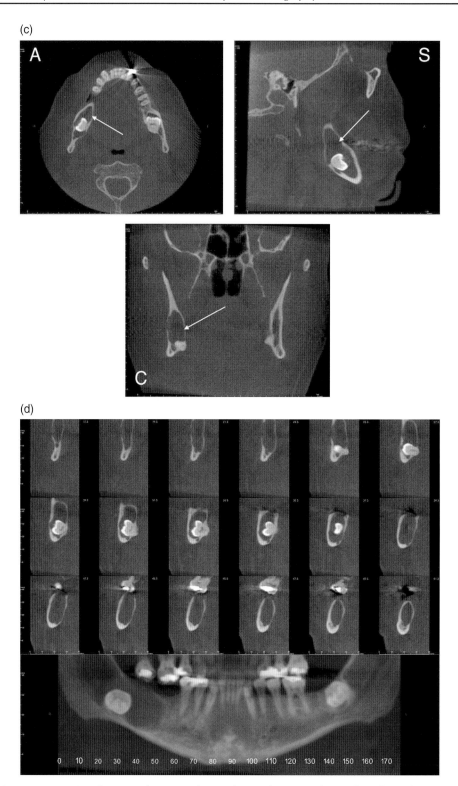

Figure 2.16. (*continued*)   (c) Axial (A), sagittal (S), and coronal (C) views showing bone loss (white arrows) in the right mandibular posterior region. (d) Reconstructed pantomograph and cross-sectional slices showing facial-lingual width of dentigerous cyst.

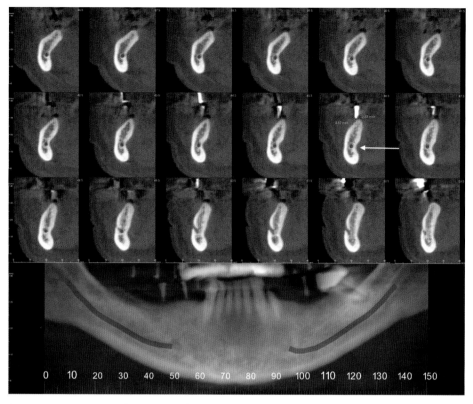

Figure 2.17.   Reconstructed pantomograph and cross-sectional slices showing lingual concavity in posterior mandible (white arrow) and mandibular canal noted in red.

Goals

Evaluate changes in alveolar bone thickness and height around natural teeth.

Benefits

CBCT aids in identifying patients undergoing orthodontic treatment who are at risk for alveolar bone/soft-tissue deficiencies.

Potential Risks

Long-term radiation hazards of effective dose accumulation are still unknown, so the practitioner should minimize exposure when possible.

Bottom Line

CBCT can assist in planning orthodontic therapy and aid in identifying those with thin bone.

Periodontitis

"Does CBCT imaging add clinical value in diagnostic assessment and treatment planning for the management of periodontitis?"

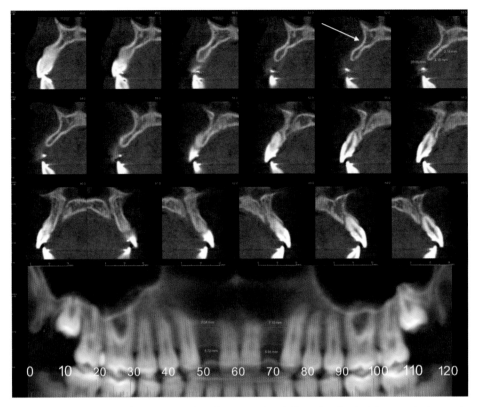

Figure 2.18.   Reconstructed pantomograph and cross-sectional slices showing facial concavity in anterior maxilla (white arrow).

Benefits

Current evidence does not support routine use of CBCT in managing periodontitis.

Potential Risks

Long-term radiation hazards of effective dose accumulation are still unknown, so the practitioner should minimize exposure when possible.

Bottom Line

CBCT provides little benefit managing periodontal disease.

References

Endodontics

AAE and AAOMR Joint Position Statement; use of cone beam computed tomography in endodontics—2015/2016 update. (https://www.aae.org/specialty/clinical-resources/guidelines-position-statements/).

Chakravarthy, P. V. K., Telang, L. A., Nerali, J., et al. (2012). Cracked tooth: A report of two cases and role of cone beam computed tomography in diagnosis. *Case Reports in Dentistry*, **2012**, 525364.

Durack, C., and Patel, S. (2012). Cone beam computed tomography in endodontics. *Braz Dent J*, **23** (3), 179–91.

Joint Position Paper AAE and AAOMR; use of cone-beam computed tomography in endodontics (http://c.ymcdn.com/sites/www.aaomr.org/resource/resmgr/Docs/AAOMR-AAE_postition_paper_CB.pdf).

Orthodontics

Clinical recommendations regarding use of cone beam computed tomography in orthodontics. Position statement by the American Academy of Oral and Maxillofacial Radiology. (https://www.aaomr.org/assets/Journal_Publications/Position_Papers/1.%20clinical%20recommendations%20%20regarding%20use%20of%20cbct%20in%20orthodontics.%20position%20statement%20by%20the%20american%20%20academy%20of%20oral%20and%20maxillofaci.pdf).

Fisher, J. (2015). Take only CBCTs on these types of orthodontic cases. *New Advances in Digital Dentistry*, **1**, 1.

Kapila, S., Conley, R. S., Harrell Jr, W. E. (2011). The current status of cone beam computed tomography imaging in orthodontics. *Dentomaxillofac Radiol*, **40** (1), 24–34.

Rossini, G., Cavallini, C., Cassetta, M., et al. (2012). Localization of impacted maxillary canines using cone beam computed tomography. Review of the literature. *Ann Stomatol (Roma)*, **3** (1), 14–8.

Periodontics

Mandelaris, G. A., Scheyer, E. T., Evans, M., et. al. (2017). American Academy of Periodontology best evidence consensus statement on selected oral applications for cone-beam computed tomography. *J Periodontol*, **88**, 939–45.

Quereshy, F. A., Barnum, G., Demko, C., et al. (2012). Use of cone beam computed tomography to volumetrically assess alveolar cleft defects—preliminary results. *J Oral Maxillofac Surg*, **70** (1), 188–91.

Tsai, P., Torabinejad, M., Rice, D., et al. (2012). Accuracy of cone-beam computed tomography and periapical radiography in detecting small periapical lesions. *J Endod*, **38**, 965–70.

Legal Issues Concerning Cone Beam Computed Tomography

Shawneen M. Gonzalez

Introduction

This chapter covers the standard of care and general recommendations about cone beam computed tomography use in dentistry. The topics covered include general recommendations from both American and European oral and maxillofacial radiological societies broken into three separate categories: prescription, use, and interpretation. Legal issues regarding cone beam computed tomography are largely recommendations to date, as there have been no major legal cases involving cone beam computed tomography as of the writing of this book. This chapter references the American legal system regarding cone beam computed tomography use.

Standard of Care

Standard of care is the base level at which a dentist must perform specific duties, including but not limited to endodontic procedures, restorative procedures, and diagnosis and treatment planning. If a health care professional performs below this level, it is considered malpractice and negligence. Violations of the standard of care can result in a loss of licensure and monetary repercussions for the dental professional.

There are two primary legal cases involving technology and standard of care: *Frye v. United States (1923)* and *Daubert v. Merrell Dow (1993)*. In 1993, the U.S. Supreme Court dismissed the *Frye* mandate that technology is admissible in court as long as it has "general acceptance" in the scientific community. Even though this ruling rejected the *Frye* mandate on a federal level, there are still several states that continue to follow *Frye's* test for admission of technology as standard of care. For those states following *Frye's* standard, an expert in the field is tapped to determine if the technology has become "general acceptance" for the field in question. The ruling

Interpretation Basics of Cone Beam Computed Tomography, Second Edition.
Edited by Shawneen M. Gonzalez.
© 2021 John Wiley & Sons, Inc. Published 2021 by John Wiley & Sons, Inc.
Companion website: www.wiley.com/go/gonzalez/interpretation

of *Daubert* determined that "scientific knowledge must be derived from the scientific method supported by good grounds in validating the expert's testimony, establishing a standard of evidentiary reliability" (Stevens 2005).

At the time of publication, cone beam computed tomography (CBCT) is not standard of care for any dental procedures in any state in the United States of America.

Recommendations

American Academy of Oral and Maxillofacial Radiology and American Dental Association Recommendations

The American Academy of Oral and Maxillofacial Radiology (AAOMR) came out with recommendation in 2008 about the use of CBCT. Since then, they have come out with more recommendations in specific areas such as implants, endodontics, orthodontics, and periodontics. This chapter will cover only the original basic recommendations, as the others are noted in Chapters 2 (specialty recommendations) and 11 (implants). The American Dental Association (ADA) came out with several recommendations about CBCT in 2012. These recommendations apply to those offices that have a CBCT unit as well as those offices that refer out for this procedure. Because there is overlap of the recommendations, I have combined them as recommendations made for the United States of America.

Prescribing a Cone Beam Computed Tomography Scan

These recommendations apply to any practitioner who prescribes a CBCT scan regardless of whether there is a unit in office.

1. Review the patient's medical and dental history along with performing a thorough clinical exam. Documentation of these procedures and justification that the excess radiation will result in a benefit outweighing the radiation risk must be included in the patient's chart prior to prescribing a scan.
2. Determine if standard 2D radiographic images show or do not show the area in question to the extent they need.
3. Have basic knowledge and education in CBCT imaging to understand what the scan will or will not show. The ADA recommends using evidence-based articles and continuing education courses to understand CBCT basics.

Use of Cone Beam Computed Tomography Scan

These recommendations apply to offices and/or imaging centers that have a CBCT unit or are planning to purchase one.

1. Prior to installing a CBCT unit in your office, a health physicist should be consulted to determine the desired location of the machine has adequate shielding based on the machine perimeters (kVp, mA, and exposure times). The health physicist will also ensure that the office is in compliance with federal and/or state radiation regulations.
2. After a CBCT unit is installed, proper training and education on safe use when performing scans must be achieved by all dental professionals who will be

operating the machine. This is typically done by the CBCT unit company. After an office is trained on safe use of a CBCT unit, it should create a quality-control program, including an evaluation interval to determine whether the machine is operating at the specified settings.

3. The CBCT unit must be operated by either a licensed practitioner or certified radiologic operator. This will be different for every state/country. In certain states and countries, a CBCT unit may be classified as a dental x-ray unit or a medical x-ray unit. For those areas where it is labeled as a dental x-ray unit, any dental professional who is legally allowed to expose a patient to radiation can operate the CBCT unit. For those areas where it is labeled as a medical x-ray unit, only a licensed radiologic technician or licensed dentist or physician may operate the machine.

4. The imaging site should always be in compliance with ALARA (as low as reasonably achievable). The office should apply this by using the smallest field of view (FOV) with the shortest exposure time to show the entire area in question. The office should also use thyroid collars and lead aprons as long as they don't interfere with the area being scanned.

5. Offices with a CBCT unit should be continually learning about CBCT and radiation safety. Technology is consistently changing, and the applications of this technology are also changing. An office must stay current to determine the best possible way to manage this new technology so as to aid in its patient care.

Interpretation of a Cone Beam Computed Tomography Scan

These recommendations apply to the interpretation of a CBCT scan.

1. The prescribing practitioner is responsible to interpret the findings of the entire scan and generate a report of the findings. The practitioner is held to the same level as a board-certified oral and maxillofacial radiologist. The scan may be interpreted by an oral and maxillofacial radiologist to aid the referring practitioner; however, the legal onus falls on the practitioner who prescribed the CBCT scan.

2. All CBCT scans should be evaluated by a dentist with training and education in CBCT interpretation. The entire captured CBCT scan must be interpreted and all findings put in the patient's chart. It is the responsibility of the prescribing practitioner to inform the patient of the findings, both normal and abnormal.

European Academy of DentoMaxilloFacial Radiology Basic Principles

In 2011, the European Academy of DentoMaxilloFacial Radiology (EADMFR) came out with 20 recommendations about CBCT use in dentistry. The recommendations, some of which are listed below, are very similar to those stated previously.

Prescribing a Cone Beam Computed Tomography Scan

1. The practitioner must review the patient's history and perform a thorough clinical exam. Documentation of these procedures and justification that the excess radiation will result in a benefit outweighing the radiation risk must be included in the patient's chart prior to prescribing a scan.

2. The practitioner should have basic knowledge of CBCT and be aware that a CBCT scan will potentially add new information and aid in the management of the patient.
3. The practitioner must use CBCT only when lower-dose traditional 2D radiography does not provide the information necessary to manage a patient.
4. A practitioner should not "routinely" prescribe CBCT scans without determining a risk/benefit for each specific scan.
5. If soft tissues are in question, conventional computed tomography (CT) or magnetic resonance imaging (MRI) should be requested instead of CBCT.

Use of Cone Beam Computed Tomography Scan

1. When a new CBCT unit is being installed in an office, it should be tested to ensure radiation protection is optimal.
2. A quality assurance program must be created for offices with a CBCT unit. The unit must be routinely tested to ensure proper radiation protection for patients and office members.
3. The guidelines in Section 6 of *Radiation Protection 136, European Guidelines on Radiation Protection in Dental Radiology* (European Academy DentoMaxilloFacial Radiology 2004) should be followed.
4. All who will be operating the CBCT unit must have theoretical and practical training in radiation protection. Continued education on CBCT and radiation protection is required. Those offices that have not received adequate training should undergo additional training involving a dentomaxillofacial radiologist.
5. The CBCT unit should have a variety of fields of view and resolution options. The smallest field of view should be used with the lowest amount of radiation necessary to capture the area in question.
6. When positioning a patient, positioning lights must be used.
7. If other practitioners refer to your office for a CBCT, they must provide you with adequate clinical information regarding the patient's history and examination.

Interpretation of a Cone Beam Computed Tomography Scan

1. All CBCT scans must have a thorough clinical evaluation (radiological report) made of the entire dataset.
2. When a CBCT scan involves the mandible and maxilla up to the floor of the nose, a radiological report should be made by a trained dentomaxillofacial radiologist or, when this is not possible, an adequately trained general dentist.
3. When a CBCT scan involves large fields of view and/or anatomy beyond the teeth and jaws, a radiological report should be made by a trained dentomaxillofacial radiologist or medical radiologist.

Summary

In summarizing this chapter, it is best to use a quote by Edwin Zinman, DDS, JDS, a California attorney, who stated in a DrBicuspid.com article, "There is no average patient. If a lesion is present on a cone-beam CT scan, then for that individual patient their statistic is 100%. Consequently, 100% of cone-beam CT scans must be diagnosed for pathosis 100% of the time by viewing 100% of cone-beam CT scanned images" (Kincade 2010).

References

American Academy of Oral and Maxillofacial Radiology. (2008). Executive opinion statement on performing and interpreting diagnostic cone beam computed tomography. *Oral Surg Oral Med Oral Pathol Oral Radiol Endod*, **106**, 561–2.

American Dental Association Council on Scientific Affairs. (2012). The use of cone beam computed tomography in dentistry; an advisory statement from the American Dental Association Council on Scientific Affairs. *JADA*, **143**, 899–902.

Curley, A., and Hatcher, D. C. (2009). Cone beam CT—anatomic assessment and legal issues: the new standards of care. *CDA Journal*, **37**, 653–62.

Daubert v. Merrell Dow Pharmaceuticals, 509 U.S. 579 (1993).

European Academy Dentomaxillofacial Radiology. Guidelines. (http://eadmfr.info/sedentexct).

European Academy Dentomaxillofacial Radiology. Radiation protection guidelines. (Ec.europa.eu/energy/nuclear/radioprotection/publication/doc/136_en.pdf).

Friedland, B. (2009). Medicolegal issues related to cone beam CT. *Semin Orthod*, **15**, 77–84.

Friedland, B., and Miles, D.A. (2014). Liabilities and risks of using cone beam computed tomography. *Dent Clin North Am*, **58**, 671–85.

Frye v. United States, 293 F. 1013 (D.C. Cir. 1923).

Kincade, K. Who is liable for incidental findings in a CBCT scan? (2010). (https://www.drbicuspid.com/index.aspx?sec=sup&sub=cad&pag=dis&ItemID=306317).

Stevens, M. 2005. Admissibility of scientific evidence under *Daubert*. (http://faculty.ncwc.edu/mstevens/425/lecture02.htm).

Zinman, E. J., White, S. C., Tetradis, S. (2010). Legal considerations in the use of cone beam computer tomography imaging. *CDA Journal*, **38** (1), 49–56.

Paranasal Sinuses and Mastoid Air Cells

Gayle Tieszen Reardon

Introduction

The paranasal sinuses of the craniofacial complex are air-filled cavities, including the maxillary sinuses, the frontal sinuses, the sphenoid sinuses, and the ethmoid air cells. The paired maxillary sinuses are of particular significance to dentistry because of the proximity of these sinuses to dental structures; in particular, the roots of the maxillary teeth. The close association of the maxillary sinuses and dental structures produces a quandary for dentists when they consider possible differential diagnoses for disease processes, which could be of either odontogenic or sinus origin. Regardless of the etiology of a specific pathologic process, the disease may spread from the dentition to sinus or from the sinus to the dentition.

With the advent of cone beam multiplanar imaging in dentistry, it is possible to visualize all paranasal sinuses on images made for dental purposes. Therefore, the dentist should be acquainted with the appearance of normal sinuses and their comparative symmetry from side to side. It is through the appreciation and knowledge of normal-appearing structures that the dentist will recognize variants of normal as well as pathology.

Anatomy

Normal Paranasal Development

The paranasal sinuses originate as evaginations from the nasal fossae into their respective bones (the maxillary bone, frontal bone, sphenoid bone, and ethmoid bone). They are lined by a mucosa that is similar to that found in the nasal cavity, which is a pseudostratified columnar ciliated epithelium containing both mucinous (goblet cells) and serous glands. Because the mucosa of the paranasal sinuses is attached directly to the bone, it is frequently referred to as mucoperiosteum. The

Interpretation Basics of Cone Beam Computed Tomography, Second Edition.
Edited by Shawneen M. Gonzalez.
© 2021 John Wiley & Sons, Inc. Published 2021 by John Wiley & Sons, Inc.
Companion website: www.wiley.com/go/gonzalez/interpretation

mucoperiosteum of the sinuses is thinner than the nasal mucosa; it is continuous with the nasal mucosa at the various sinus ostia (Figures 4.1–4.16; Table 4.1).

The functional reason for paranasal sinus presence has been discussed since the early descriptions of the sinuses in the 1800s. Proposed functions have included

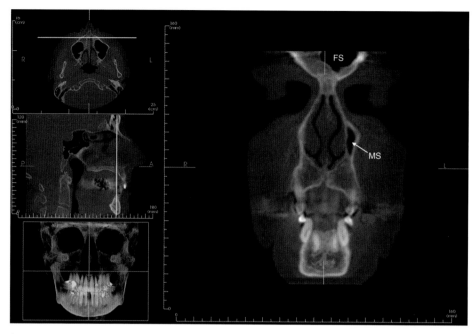

Figure 4.1. Coronal view showing the left frontal sinus (FS) and left maxillary sinus (MS). Yellow line showing coronal plane on left views (axial and sagittal).

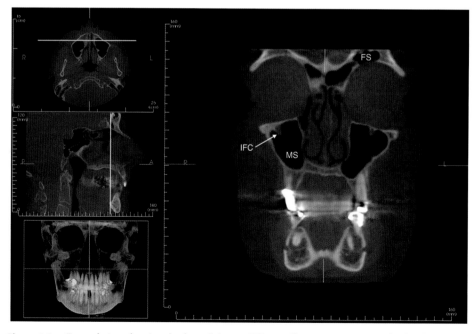

Figure 4.2. Coronal view showing the frontal sinuses (FS), maxillary sinuses (MS), and infraorbital canal (IFC). Yellow line showing coronal plane on left views (axial and sagittal).

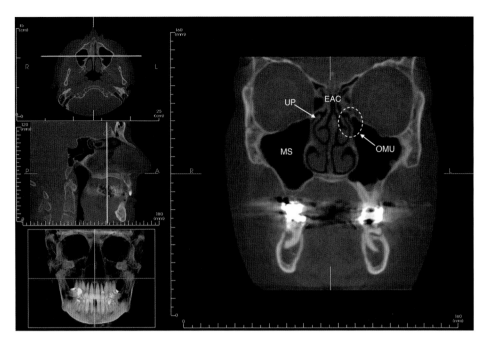

Figure 4.3. Coronal view showing the ethmoid air cells (EAC), ostiomeatal unit (OMU), uncinate process (UP), and maxillary sinuses (MS). Yellow line showing coronal plane on left views (axial and sagittal).

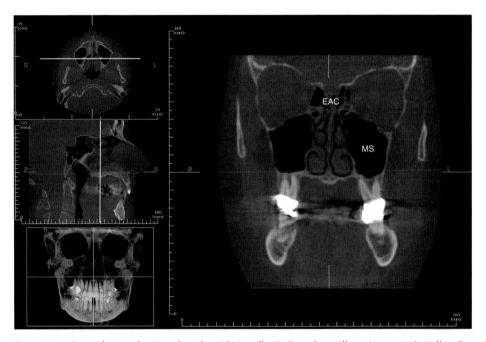

Figure 4.4. Coronal view showing the ethmoid air cells (EAC) and maxillary sinuses (MS). Yellow line showing coronal plane on left views (axial and sagittal).

contributing to voice resonance, the humidification and warmth of inspired air, to increase the olfactory membrane area, to absorb shock to the face and head, to provide thermal insulation for the brain, to lighten the skull and facial bones, and to contribute to facial growth. The current documented thought is that the paranasal sinuses form a collapsible framework, which helps to protect the brain from blunt trauma.

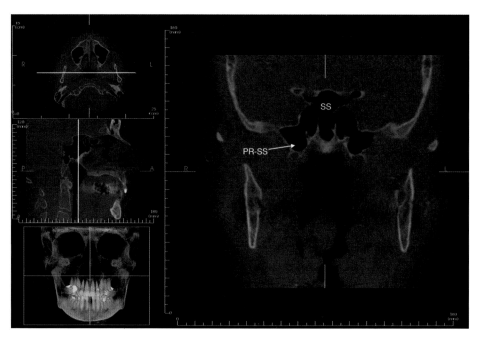

Figure 4.5.   Coronal view showing the sphenoid sinuses (SS) with bilateral pterygoid recess of the sphenoid sinus (PR-SS). Yellow line showing coronal plane on left views (axial and sagittal).

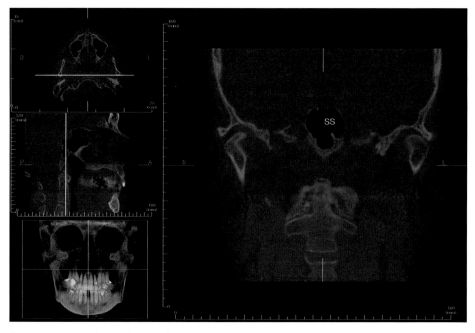

Figure 4.6.   Coronal view showing the posterior aspect of the sphenoid sinuses (SS). Yellow line showing coronal plane on left views (axial and sagittal).

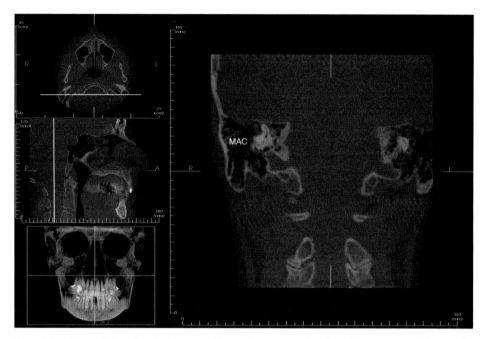

Figure 4.7. Coronal view showing the mastoid air cells (MAC). Yellow line showing coronal plane on left views (axial and sagittal).

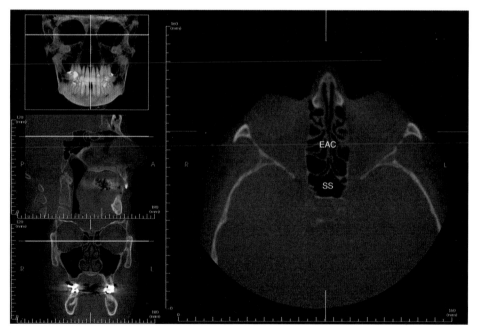

Figure 4.8. Axial view showing the ethmoid air cells (EAC) and sphenoid sinuses (SS). Yellow line showing axial plane on left views (3D reconstruction, sagittal, and coronal).

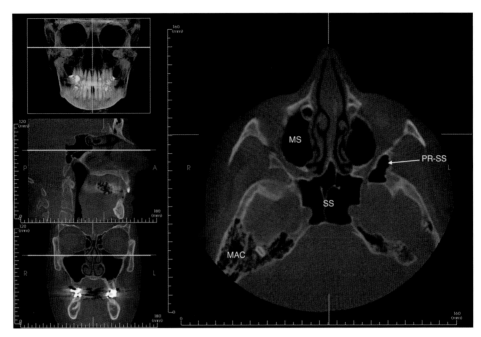

Figure 4.9.   Axial view showing the maxillary sinuses (MS), sphenoid sinuses (SS), pteryboid recess of the sphenoid sinus (PR-SS), and mastoid air cells (MAC). Yellow line showing axial plane on left views (3D reconstruction, sagittal, and coronal).

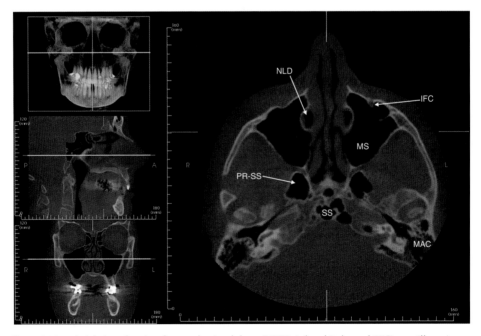

Figure 4.10.   Axial view showing the nasolacrimal ducts (NLD), infraorbital canal (IFC), maxillary sinuses (MS), bilateral pterygoid recess of the sphenoid sinuses (PR-SS), sphenoid sinuses (SS), and mastoid air cells (MAC). Yellow line showing axial plane on left views (3D reconstruction, sagittal, and coronal).

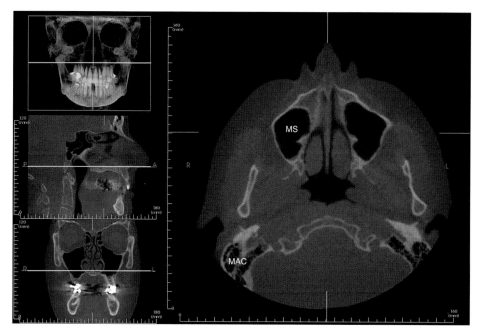

Figure 4.11. Axial view showing the maxillary sinuses (MS) and mastoid air cells (MAC). Yellow line showing axial plane on left views (3D reconstruction, sagittal, and coronal).

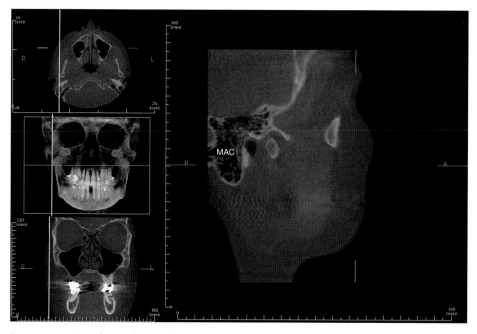

Figure 4.12. Sagittal view showing the mastoid air cells (MAC). Yellow line showing sagittal plane on left views (axial, 3D reconstruction, and coronal).

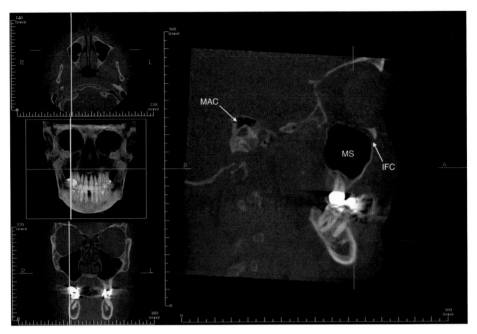

Figure 4.13. Sagittal view showing mastoid air cells (MAC), maxillary sinus (MS), and infraorbital canal (IFC). Yellow line showing sagittal plane on left views (axial, 3D reconstruction, and coronal).

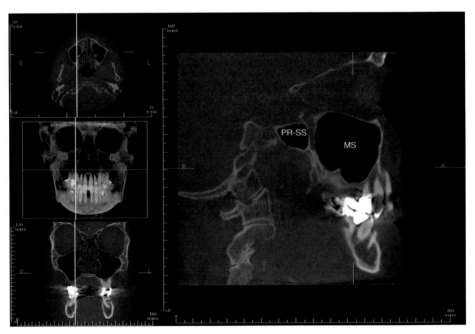

Figure 4.14. Sagittal view showing the maxillary sinus (MS) and a pterygoid recess of the sphenoid sinus (PR-SS). Yellow line showing sagittal plane on left views (axial, 3D reconstruction, and coronal).

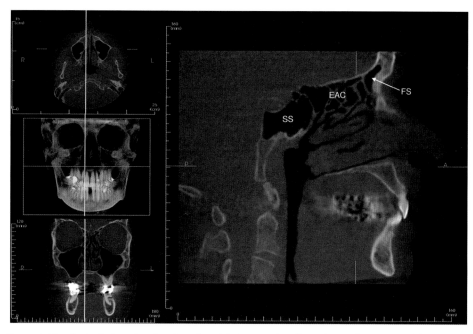

Figure 4.15. Sagittal view showing the sphenoid sinuses (SS), ethmoid air cells (EAC), and frontal sinus (FS). Yellow line showing sagittal plane on left views (axial, 3D reconstruction and coronal).

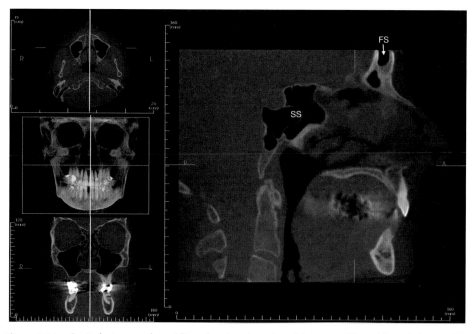

Figure 4.16. Sagittal view on the midline showing the sphenoid sinuses (SS) and frontal sinuses (FS). Yellow line showing sagittal plane on left views (axial, 3D reconstruction, and coronal).

Table 4.1.   Anatomical landmarks identifiable in corresponding figures.

Anatomical landmark	Coronal	Axial	Sagittal
Frontal sinus (FS)	4.1 4.2		4.15 4.16
Ethmoid air cells (EAC)	4.3 4.4	4.8	4.15
Maxillary sinus (MS)	4.1 4.2 4.3 4.4	4.9 4.10 4.11	4.13 4.14
Infraorbital canal (IFC)	4.2	4.10	4.13
Sphenoid sinus (SS)	4.5 4.6	4.8 4.9 4.10	4.15 4.16
Pterygoid recess of sphenoid sinus (PR-SS)	4.5	4.9 4.10	4.14
Mastoid air cells (MAC)	4.7	4.9 4.10 4.11	4.12 4.13

Maxillary Sinus

The maxillary sinus is the first of the paranasal sinuses to form and is visualized by the 70th day of gestation. After each nasal fossa and its turbinates are established, a small ridge develops just above the inferior turbinate, marking the future uncinate process. Shortly thereafter, an evagination above this ridge, the uncibullous groove, is seen, which enlarges laterally from the nasal cavity and is the site of the original maxillary sinus bud. These early evaginations continue their growth laterally beneath the orbits through a process of pneumatization, which occurs concurrent to the growth of the maxilla and alveolar process. By birth, the rudimentary maxillary sinus appears like a small slit lying just medial to the orbit. The size of the neonate's maxillary sinus is approximately 7 × 4 × 4 mm, with the longest dimension being the anteroposterior axis.

The annual growth rate of the maxillary sinus is approximately 2 mm vertically and 3 mm anteroposteriorly. By the end of year 1, the lateral margin extends under the medial portion of the orbit. By 2 years of age, the sinus extends laterally to the infraorbital canal and passes inferolaterally to it during years 3 and 4. At 9 years, the maxillary sinus extends laterally to the zygomatic bone and is near level with the floor of the nasal fossa. Lateral growth of the maxillary sinuses continues until mid-adolescence, approximately 15 years of age. The final descent of the sinus, an indicator of sinus growth cessation, is not complete until the third molar has erupted. By adulthood, the average volume of the maxillary sinus is approximately 14.75 ml and its mean dimensions are 34 mm deep, 33 mm high, and 25 mm wide. The average adult maxillary sinus volume is approximately 14.75 ml.

Generally speaking, the maxillary sinuses develop quite symmetrically and may continue to enlarge or pneumatize throughout life through the formation of air cells or cavities in tissues and adjacent bony structures. However, hypoplasia of the maxilla resulting from trauma, infection, surgical intervention, or irradiation to the developing maxilla can damage maxillary growth centers, producing a small maxilla and a hypoplastic sinus. Hypoplastic sinuses are also seen in Treacher Collins syndrome, mandibulofacial dysostosis, and thalassemia major due to brachial arch anomalies when the demand for marrow prohibits sinus pneumatization.

The floor of the maxillary sinus is lowest near the second premolar and first molar teeth, lying 3–5 mm below the nasal floor. The roots of the first, second, and third molars form conical elevations that project into the floor of the sinus. Less often, the roots of the premolar teeth and, more rarely, the canine teeth project into the antrum. The expansion of the maxillary sinus antrum is closely related to dentition. When a tooth erupts, the vacated space becomes pneumatized, which then serves to expand the sinus lumen.

The infraorbital, greater palatine, posterosuperior alveolar, and anterosuperior alveolar arteries, all branches of the maxillary artery, contribute to the blood supply of the maxillary sinus. Additionally, the sphenopalatine artery's lateral branches and a small branch of the facial artery contribute to the antrum's blood supply.

The nerve supply of the antrum is through branches of the second division of the trigeminal nerve, specifically the branches of the superior alveolar nerves, the anterior palatine nerve, and the infraorbital nerve. It is the posterior superior alveolar nerve that pierces the posterior wall of the antrum, running forward and downward to supply the molar teeth.

Normal Anatomy of the Ostiomeatal Complex

Given the fact that sinusitis, or sinusoidal inflammatory disease, is a serious health problem affecting between 30 and 50 million people in the United States alone, it is obvious that correct interpretation of sinus imaging studies is of paramount importance. Therefore, it is important to understand the anatomy of the ostiomeatal complex. The definition of the ostiomeatal complex is: *The point in the middle meatus where the frontal and maxillary sinuses normally drain into the nasal cavity; obstruction here predisposes inflammation and infection of affected sinus cavities.*

The ostiomeatal complex, known also as the ostiomeatal unit, consists of the lateral nasal wall and its adjacent structures (Figure 4.17). It is the lateral nasal wall that contains the bulbous projections known as the turbinates (concha), which are divided into three levels: superior, middle, and inferior turbinates. Occasionally, there is a fourth level of concha called supreme, which is above the superior concha. The superior meatus drains the posterior ethmoid air cells and, more posteriorly, the sphenoid sinuses via the sphenoethmoidal recess. The middle meatus receives drainage from the frontal sinus, the maxillary sinus, and the anterior ethmoid air cells. The recesses draining each of these three regions of the paranasal sinuses are as follows:

1. The frontal sinus is drained via the frontal recess.
2. The maxillary sinus is drained via the maxillary ostium and, subsequently, the ethmoidal infundibulum.
3. The anterior ethmoid air cells are drained via the ethmoid air cell ostia.

(a)

(b)

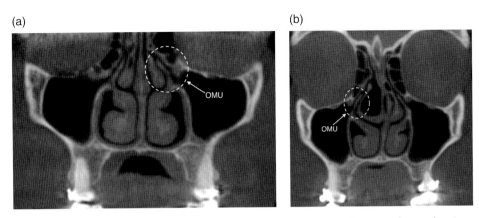

Figure 4.17. (a) Coronal view showing a patent ostiomeatal unit (OMU). (b) Coronal view showing a patent ostiomeatal unit (OMU).

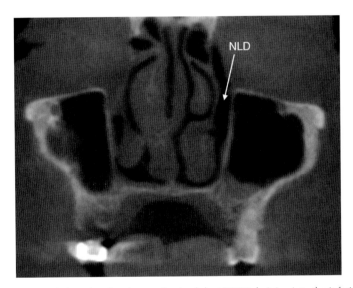

Figure 4.18. Coronal view showing the nasolacrimal duct (NLD) draining into the inferior meatus.

The nasolacrimal duct is drained via the inferior meatus (Figure 4.18).

Morphological evaluation in this region must focus upon the anatomy adjacent to these structures that contributes to constrictions in this region. It is the anatomical "tight spots" or constrictions that create drainage challenges contributing to sinusitis. If potential constrictions are considered by area, the first site encountered is in the anterior region surrounding the frontal recess, followed by the area surrounding the infundibulum and the middle meatus, and, finally, the most posteriorly situated region involving the sphenoethmoid recess.

When observing sinus anatomy on medical computed tomography (CT) or cone beam computed tomography (CBCT), one will quickly observe there is central septation dividing the right side from the left side. While this left/right division is the most obvious, it should be noted there may be several levels of septation, and the floor of the frontal sinus slopes inferiorly toward the midline, an arrangement that is very complementary to the frontal sinuses' overall funnel shape.

(a) (b)

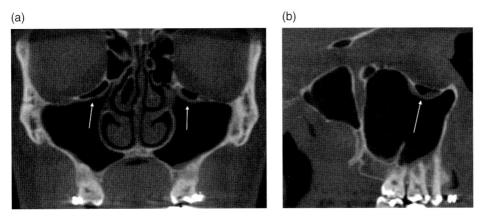

Figure 4.19.   (a) Coronal view showing bilateral Haller cells (white arrows) inferior to the orbital cavity. (b) Sagittal view showing Haller cell (white arrow) with mucosal thickening at the superior surface of the maxillary sinus.

Starting at the superior aspect of the ostiomeatal unit is the frontal recess, which is hourglass shaped, narrowing between the frontal sinuses and the anterior middle meatus. It is the frontal recess that drains the frontal sinus. The frontal recess is not a tubular or ductlike structure. Rather, it is a recess, as the term *nasofrontal recess* (also referred to as the nasofrontal duct) would imply. The nasofrontal recess is the primary ostium located in the depression in the floor of the frontal sinus.

Anterior, lateral, and inferior to the frontal recess and at the supero-medial aspect of the orbit is the agger nasi cell, which is a remnant ethmoturbinal cell present in nearly all patients. The agger nasi cell represents the most anterior ethmoid air cell lying deep within the lacrimal bone. It is the size of the agger nasi cell that determines the patency of the frontal recess and the anterior middle meatus. When considering the anterior air channels, it is noteworthy to observe that the frontal recess is the narrowest and thus a common site for inflammation. Obstruction of the agger nasi cell decreases ventilation and mucociliary clearance from the frontal sinus.

There are several anatomical variations that may cause obstruction of the anterior ostiomeatal unit, including deviation of the nasal septum, presence of infraorbital ethmoid cells (Haller cells; Figure 4.19), and variations in the size and shape of the ethmoid air bulla, middle turbinate, uncinate process, and frontal cells.

Ethmoid Sinuses

The ethmoid sinuses, also known as the ethmoid air cells, occupy the space between the frontal and sphenoidal sinuses. The paired ethmoidal cell groups bulge into the upper portion of the nasal fossa and have ostia that drain into the adjacent middle and superior meatus. The ethmoidal sinuses are divided into groups of cells by bony basal lamellae that extend laterally to the laminae papyracea and superiorly to the fovea ethmoidalis. These five lamellae serve as attachments for the turbinates, one for each of the primary turbinates (middle, superior, and, when present, supreme) and one for each of the secondary turbinates (bullae ethmoidalis and uncinate process).

The ethmoidal sinuses begin their formation in the third to fifth fetal months of life when numerous separate evaginations arise from the nasal cavity. The anterior cells are the first to form as evaginations in the lateral nasal wall in the region of the middle meatus. Development of the posterior cells follows as evaginations in the superior meatal area. During the fifth prenatal month of life, the ethmoid air cells have expanded into the ethmoid bones and continue their expansion until puberty, or until the sinus walls reach a layer of compact bone, which halts enlargement. While the lamellae prevent one group of cells from intermingling with another, they do not prevent intramural expansion of one group into another. A concha bullosa results when posterior ethmoid cells extend intramurally to pneumatize the middle turbinate. This can result in a large obstructing turbinate or a focus of infection.

At birth, the anterior ethmoidal complex is about 5 mm high, 2 mm long, and 2 mm wide. The posterior cell group is 5 mm high, 4 mm long, and 2 mm wide. The sinuses reach their adult size by the age of 12 years. The adult ethmoid has between 3 and 18 cells. The number of ethmoid air cells varies per side with each containing between 8 and 15 chambers. As with the maxillary sinuses, the ethmoid air cells may extend into neighboring bony structures of the maxillary, lacrimal, frontal, sphenoid, and palatine bones.

The ethmoid sinuses receive their blood supply from the nasal branches of the sphenopalatine artery and from the anterior and posterior ethmoidal arteries, which are branches of the ophthalmic artery. The sensory innervation of the ethmoid mucosa is via the ophthalmic and maxillary divisions of the trigeminal nerve. The anterior cells are supplied by the nasociliary branch of the ophthalmic division via the anterior ethmoidal nerve. The posterior ethmoidal cells are supplied by the posterior ethmoidal nerve from the ophthalmic division and the posterolateral nasal branches of the sphenopalatine nerve from the maxillary division of the trigeminal nerve.

Frontal Sinus

The frontal sinuses arise from one of several outgrowths originating in the region of the frontal recess of the nose or from anterior ethmoid cells of the infundibulum. Their site of origin can be identified on the mucosa as early as 3–4 months *in utero*. The frontal sinuses are absent at birth, with their delayed development starting after the second year of life. They reach the frontal bone around the fifth or sixth year of childhood. The frontal sinuses are essentially displaced anterior ethmoid cells, and because they develop from a variable site, their drainage will be either via an ostium into the frontal recess or via a nasofrontal duct into the anterior ethmoidal infundibulum.

Approximately 4% of the population will fail to develop frontal sinuses. On average, the cranial extent of the frontal sinus is half the height of the orbit by the age of 4 years. By 8 years of age, the top of the frontal sinuses is at the level of the orbital roof. At age 10, the sinuses extend into the vertical portion of the frontal bone. Their adult size is reached after puberty.

Each frontal sinus develops separately on the right and left sides of the frontal bone and grows toward the midline. Often the larger sinus extends across the midsagittal plane and appears to be somewhat centered. The frontal sinuses are asymmetric in shape, and their size is widely variable. In spite of the wide variability in frontal sinus size, the average frontal sinus has been described as between 28 mm high, 24 mm wide, and 20 mm deep. A direct relationship between the mechanical stresses of mastication and frontal sinus enlargement has been demonstrated, as has a direct relationship with growth hormone, as seen in acromegaly.

Because of its variable origin, about 40% of frontal sinuses drain into the ethmoidal infundibulum. In these cases, the ethmoidal infundibulum acts as a channel carrying secretions from the frontal sinus to the anterior ethmoidal cells and maxillary sinus, or vice versa. The natural frontal sinus ostium is usually located in the posteromedial floor of the sinus.

The main arterial supply to the frontal sinus is via the supraorbital and supratrochlear arteries, both of which are derived from the ophthalmic artery. The sensory innervation of the sinus mucosa is via the supraorbital and supratrochlear branches of the frontal nerve, which is a branch of the first division of the trigeminal nerve.

Sphenoid Sinus

The sphenoid sinuses emerge in the fourth month *in utero* as evaginations from the posterior nasal capsule into the sphenoid bone. This occurs above small crescent-shaped ridges of bone, the sphenoidal conchae, that project from the undersurface of the body of the sphenoid bone. These conchae grow anteriorly, fusing with the posterior ethmoid labyrinth. It is rare for the sphenoid sinuses to be completely absent. However, the extent of their pneumatization varies considerably.

Emerging as diminutive spaces in the body of the neonatal sphenoid bone, the sphenoid sinuses remain small; major growth begins in the third to fifth year of life. By the age of 7 years, the sinus has extended posteriorly to the level of the anterior sella turcica wall. By 10–12 years of age, the sinus has achieved its adult configuration. Absence of sphenoid sinus pneumatization by age 10 years is suggestive of "occult" sphenoid bone pathology consistent with diseases requiring a large marrow demand to compensate for chronic anemia, such as thalassemia and chronic renal failure.

Like the maxillary and frontal sinuses, the sphenoid sinuses are a paired sinus with asymmetric right and left sides. The two sides are separated by a bony septum. The average adult sphenoid sinus is 20 mm high, 23 mm long, and 17 mm wide. The degree of sphenoid sinus pneumatization is classified as nonpneumatized, presellar or sellar. The sphenoid sinuses communicate with the nasal cavities through ostia that are usually 2–3 mm in diameter.

The arterial supply of the sphenoid sinus is from branches of both the internal and external carotid arteries. The posterior ethmoidal branch of the ophthalmic artery may contribute vessels to the roof of the sphenoid sinus, and the floor of the sinus receives blood from the sphenopalatine branch of the maxillary artery. The sphenoid sinus is innervated by both the second and third divisions of the trigeminal nerve.

Onodi Cells

The literature presents two alternative definitions for "Onodi cells." The view is the Onodi cells are actually the most posterior ethmoid cells located superolateral to the sphenoid sinus and closely associated with the optic nerve. The other definition describes Onodi cells as posterior ethmoid cells extending into the sphenoid bone, situated either adjacent to or impinging upon the optic nerve (Figure 4.20).

(a)   (b)

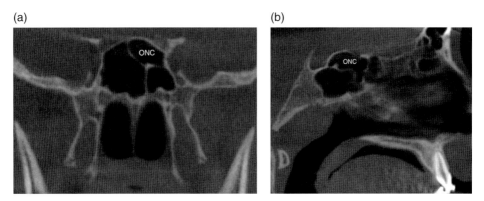

Figure 4.20.   (a) Coronal view showing Onodi cell (ONC) superior to the left sphenoid sinus. (b) Sagittal view showing Onodi cell (ONC) superior to the left sphenoid sinus.

Frontal Cells

The superior extension of the lateral nasal wall, which is also the medial wall of the maxillary sinus, is called the uncinate process. The agger nasi cell, the posteromedial wall of the nasolacrimal duct, and the uncinate process are fused anteriorly leaving the superoposterior edge of the uncinate process "free." The infundibulum is an air passageway connecting the maxillary sinus ostium with the middle meatus. The ethmoid bulla is posterior to the uncinate process; the ethmoid bullae are generally the largest of the anterior ethmoid cells (Figure 4.21). The uncinate process courses medially and inferiorly to the ethmoid bulla, which is enclosed laterally by the lamina papyracea medial to the orbit. The lamina papyracea by definition is a thin plate of ethmoidal bone forming part of the medial wall of the orbit and the lateral wall for the ethmoidal labyrinth.

There is a space between the ethmoid bulla and the free edge of the uncinate process, which delineates the hiatus semilunaris. The hiatus semilunaris communicates medially with the middle meatus, the air space lateral to the middle concha.

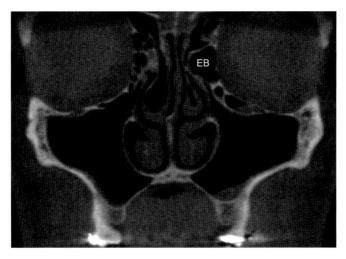

Figure 4.21.   Coronal view showing a left ethmoid bulla (EB).

The hiatus semilunaris also communicates inferolaterally with the infundibulum, the air passageway between the uncinate process and the inferomedial margin of the orbit. Primary drainage for the maxillary sinus is through the infundibulum.

The middle concha is medial to the ethmoid bulla and uncinate process. It attaches to the medial wall of the agger nasi cell anteriorly as well as the superior edge of the uncinate process. Superiorly, the middle concha adheres to the lateral aspect of the cribriform plate. The middle concha is the source of several posterolaterally coursing bony structures known as "lateral fanning" attachments, which extend to the lamina papyracea. The first of these lateral fanning attachments is the basal lamella situated posterior to the ethmoid bulla. The basal lamella separates the anterior ethmoid air cells from the posterior ethmoid air cells. In most patients, the posterior wall of the ethmoid bulla remains intact with an air passage, the sinus lateralis now known as the retrobullar recess cell, coursing between the basal lamella and the posterior ethmoid bulla and communicating with the frontal recess.

Embedded in the clivus and bordered superoposteriorly by sella turcica, the sphenoid sinus is the most posterior sinus. The ostium for the sphenoid sinus is located mediosuperiorly in the anterior sinus wall and communicates with the sphenoethmoidal recess and posterior aspect of the superior meatus. The nasal septum lies medial to the sphenoethmoidal recess.

All septations in the sphenoid sinuses are vertically oriented. Of particular importance are septations that adhere to the bony canal wall covering the internal carotid artery, which may project into the posterolateral sphenoid sinus. The vidian nerve and the second division of cranial nerve V are other structures projecting into the floor of the sphenoid sinuses. These and all other significant structures of the paranasal sinuses including the anterior cranial fossa, the cribriform plate, the cavernous sinuses, the orbits, and the optic nerves must be observed by surgeons to avoid potential postoperative complications.

Pneumatic Cells of the Temporal Bone: The Mastoid Air Cells

The air cells of the temporal bone develop as outpouchings of the antrum, epitympanum, tympanic cavity, and Eustachian tube. Tentative epithelial evaginations appear from the antrum as early as 34 weeks but there is no significant pneumatic cellular expansion into the remainder of the temporal bone until after birth. The expansion occurring after birth occurs with stimulation brought about by the presence of air within the middle ear. The pneumatization process ramps up to a high level of activity and proceeds over a period of several years. The petrous apex shows continuing pneumatization into early adulthood. The pneumatizing process occurs as a result of epithelium-lined projections arising from the lining of the middle ear and its extensions. These evaginations probe the spaces between new bone spicules and degenerating bone marrow spaces. The air cells invade the bone after the marrow has been converted into loose mesenchymal tissue. The presence of middle ear infections in infancy causes embryonic subepithelial connective tissue to fibrose, thus impeding the progress of the advancing fingers of evaginating pneumatic cells.

The mastoid process begins its development during the second year of life with downward growth of the squamous portion and partially as a result of extension of the petrous portion of the temporal bone. These two portions of the mastoid process come together at the petrosquamous suture line. Air cells grow down from the antrum vertically toward the mastoid tip and laterally and radially into the squamous portion. Koerner's septum is a dividing bridge of bone that separates these two cell tracks at the junction of the petrous and mastoid ossifications. Koerner's septum is visible radiographically as a pointed bony spicule originating from the antral roof and directed obliquely inferiorly.

The mastoid air cells are a section of the mastoid process of the temporal bone of the cranium that are hollowed out into a number of spaces. These spaces exhibit great variety in size and number. At the anterosuperior portion of the process, the cells are large and irregular and contain air, but toward the lower part of the process, they diminish in size. Those cells at the apex of the process are frequently quite small and contain marrow. Occasionally, the air cells are entirely absent, and the mastoid bone is solid throughout.

Inflammatory Disease of the Paranasal Sinuses

Inflammation may result from a variety of causes, including infection, chemical irritation, allergies, the introduction of a foreign body, or facial trauma. Imaging changes associated with inflammation include thickening of the sinus mucosa, development of an air-fluid level in the sinus(es), polyps, empyema, and retention pseudocysts. Viral infections may not trigger a radiographic change in the involved sinus(s).

Cone beam computed tomography (CBCT) is becoming increasingly more important in the evaluation of sinus disease and is an acceptable substitute for the significantly higher radiation modality, conventional computed tomography (CT). Because CBCT provides multiple viewing planes and slices through the paranasal sinuses, it may be useful for determining the differential diagnosis of sinus pathology by making it possible to outline the perimeters of the disease process. Axial and coronal CBCT examinations are the most useful noninvasive techniques for diagnosis of pathology of the paranasal sinuses and adjacent structures. CBCT examination is appropriate to determine the extent of disease in patients who have chronic or recurrent sinusitis. Coronal CBCT provides visualization of the ostiomeatal complexes and nasal cavities and demonstrates reaction of the surrounding bone to sinus pathology.

Mucositis

Definition/Clinical Characteristics

Mucositis is a thickening of the mucous membrane of the paranasal sinuses. This mucosal lining, normally about 1 mm thick, is made up of respiratory epithelium, which is not normally visualized on radiographic images. However, when the mucosa becomes irritated and inflamed from either an infectious or allergic process, its thickness may increase by 10–15 times, making visualization of the thickened membrane possible. Mucositis is the change in the thickness of the mucous membrane brought about by inflammation. Mucosal thickening greater than 3 mm is likely pathologic.

(a)   (b)

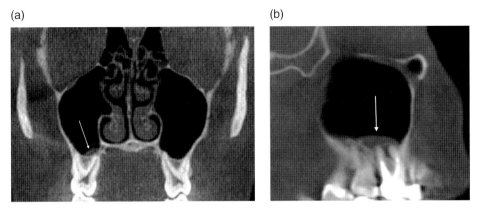

Figure 4.22.   (a) Coronal view showing minimal thickening of the mucosal lining in the right maxillary sinus consistent with mucositis (white arrow). (b) Sagittal view showing minimal thickening of the mucosal lining in the right maxillary sinus consistent with mucositis (white arrow).

Radiographic Description

The appearance of mucositis is that of a minimally thickened noncorticated radiopaque band. It is more radiopaque than the adjacent air-filled sinus. The somewhat thickened band parallels the bony wall of the affected sinus (Figures 4.22 and 4.23).

Differential Interpretation

There are no differential interpretations based on the location and appearance of this finding.

Treatment/Recommendations

No further imaging or treatment is recommended.

Sinusitis

Sinusitis is a condition involving generalized inflammation of the paranasal sinus mucosa. The etiologic agent may be an allergen, bacterial, or viral. Sinusitis may impede drainage from the ostiomeatal complex. Inflammatory changes may lead to ciliary dysfunction and retention of sinus secretions. It is estimated that approximately 10% of inflammatory episodes of the maxillary sinuses are secondary extensions of dental infections. Sinusitis may be classified into commonly used subtypes based on length of time the disease has been present.

Acute Sinusitis

Definition/Clinical Characteristics/Radiographic Description

An acute sinusitis is usually due to bacterial infection of an obstructed paranasal sinus. The obstruction is often the result of apposition of edematous mucosal surfaces from an antecedent viral upper respiratory tract infection. The edematous mucosa disrupts

(a)

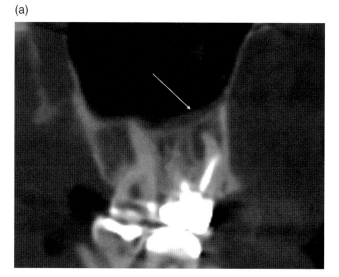

(b)

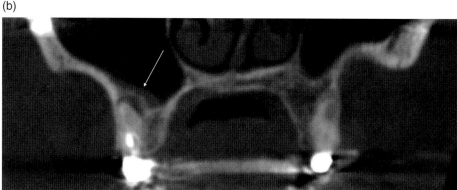

Figure 4.23.   (a) Sagittal view showing minimal thickening of the mucosal lining (white arrow) of the right maxillary sinus superior to apical rarefying osteitis of the first molar. (b) Coronal view showing minimal thickening of the mucosal lining (white arrow) of the right maxillary sinus superior to apical rarefying osteitis of the first molar.

the normal mucociliary drainage pattern of the sinus, resulting in obstruction of the sinus ostium. This obstruction of the ostium alters the oxygen tension within the obstructed sinus and predisposes the sinus to a bacterial superinfection.

Acute sinusitis refers to a condition present for a short time, generally less than 2 weeks. It usually involves only a single sinus, with the ethmoid sinus being the most common location. Acute maxillary sinusitis, often a complication of the common cold, is accompanied by a clear nasal discharge or pharyngeal drainage (Figures 4.24 and 4.25). After a few days, the stuffiness and nasal discharge increase, and the patient may complain of pain and tenderness to pressure over the involved sinus.

Differential Interpretation/Treatment/Recommendations

The pain may also be referred to the premolar and/or molar teeth on the affected side and may produce tooth sensitivity to percussion. When there is tooth tenderness to percussion, the dentist must rule out odontogenic inflammation as the possible source of pain and/or infection.

(a) (b)

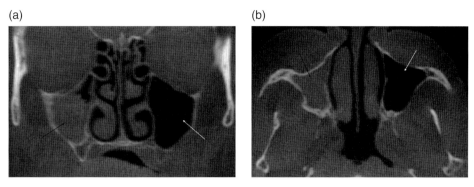

Figure 4.24. (a) Coronal view showing partial radiopacification of the right maxillary sinus (black arrow) compared to the air-filled left maxillary sinus (white arrow). (b) Axial view showing radiopacification of the right maxillary sinus (black arrow) compared to the air-filled left maxillary sinus (white arrow).

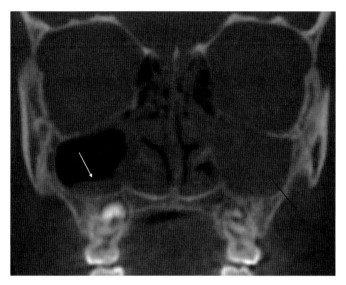

Figure 4.25. Coronal view showing radiopacification of the left maxillary sinus (black arrow) with soft-tissue thickening of the right maxillary sinus (white arrow) consistent with sinusitis.

Chronic Sinusitis

Definition/Clinical Characteristics/Radiographic Description

"Chronic sinusitis" is diagnosed when the patient has repeated bouts of acute infection or persistent inflammation commonly due to staphylococcus, streptococcus, corynebacteria, bacteroides, fusobacteria, and other anaerobes. Anaerobes are more frequently involved in chronic sinusitis than in acute sinusitis. The sinuses most commonly involved with chronic sinusitis are the anterior ethmoid air cells.

Opacification of the ostiomeatal unit has been found to predispose patients to sinusitis. In chronic sinusitis, the inflammation may stimulate the periosteum of the sinus to produce bone, resulting in thickened sclerotic borders of the maxillary sinus (Figure 4.26). Chronic sinusitis is often associated with anatomic derangements that inhibit mucous outflow, such as deviated nasal septum and the presence of a concha bullosa (pneumatization of the middle concha).

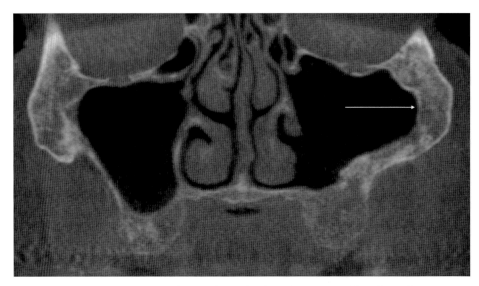

Figure 4.26.   Coronal view showing thickened bone border (white arrow) of the left maxillary sinus consistent with a history of chronic sinusitis.

Differential Interpretation/Treatment/Recommendations

Chronic sinusitis may also be associated with allergic rhinitis, asthma, cystic fibrosis, and dental infections. Referral to an ear, nose, and throat physician or a primary physician is recommended.

Fungal Sinusitis

Definition/Clinical Characteristics/Radiographic Description

Fungal sinusitis may be suspected when the patient fails to respond to standard antibiotic therapy. According to Som and Curtin (2003), the presence of fungal infection is suggested when soft-tissue changes present with thickened reactive bone with localized areas of osteomyelitis and the association of inflammatory sinus disease with involvement of the adjacent nasal fossa and soft tissues of the neck. These signs of aggressive infection are atypical of bacterial pathogens of the sinus.

Allergic Sinusitis

Definition/Clinical Characteristics/Radiographic Description

Allergic sinusitis occurs in 10% of the population and typically produces a pansinusitis with symmetric involvement. CT often shows a nodular mucosal thickening with thickened turbinates; air-fluid levels (Figure 4.27) are rare unless bacterial superinfection occurs.

Intrinsic Disease of the Paranasal Sinuses

The most common radiopaque patterns that occur in the coronal CT view are localized mucosal thickenings along the floor of the sinus, generalized thickening of the mucosal lining around the entire wall of the sinus, and near-complete or complete

(a)

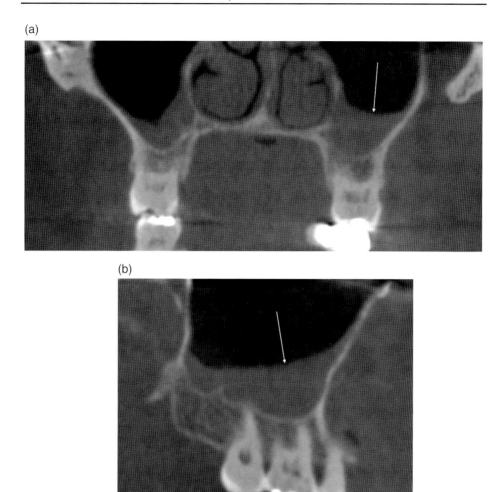

(b)

Figure 4.27. (a) Coronal view showing an air-fluid level (white arrow) of the left maxillary sinus. (b) Sagittal view showing an air-fluid level (white arrow) of the left maxillary sinus.

opacification of the sinus as seen in "silent sinus." Such changes are best seen in the maxillary sinuses, but the frontal and sphenoid sinuses may produce a similar appearance.

Scrutinizing the area around the maxillary ostium on the coronal views of CT and CBCT images may reveal the presence of thickened mucosal tissue, which may cause blockage of the ostium. Mucosal thickening in just the base of the sinus may not represent sinusitis. Rather, it may represent the more localized thickening that can occur in association with apical rarefying osteitis from a tooth with a nonvital pulp. However, this may, over time, progress to involve the entire sinus.

The inability to perceive the delicate walls of the ethmoid air cells is a sign of ethmoid sinusitis. The image of thickened sinus mucosa on CT may be uniform or polypoid. In the case of an allergic reaction, the mucosa tends to be more lobulated. In cases of sinus infection, the thickened mucosa tends to be smoother, with contours following the sinus wall.

The goal of sinusitis is to control the infection by promoting drainage, which will then relieve pain. Acute sinusitis is usually treated over the counter or prescribed decongestants to reduce mucosal swelling and, in cases of bacterial sinusitis, with antibiotics. As stated above, chronic sinusitis is generally a disease of ostia obstruction. Therefore, the goal is to drain and ventilate through means such as endoscopic surgery to enlarge obstructed ostia or establish an alternate path for drainage.

Retention Pseudocyst

Definition/Clinical Characteristics

Retention pseudocysts are known by many names, including the following: antral pseudocyst, benign mucous cyst, mucous retention cyst, mucous retention pseudocyst, mesothelial cyst, pseudocyst, interstitial cyst, lymphangiectatic cyst, false cyst, retention cyst of the maxillary sinus, benign cyst of the antrum, benign mucosal cyst of the sinus, serous nonsecretory retention pseudocyst, and mucosal antral cyst.

Retention pseudocyst is a term used to describe several related conditions with controversial etiologies but clinical and radiographic similarities. One explanation suggests that seromucous gland secretory duct blockage results in a pathologic submucosal secretion accumulation, producing swelling of the tissue. A second possibility for serous nonsecretory retention cyst formation suggests there is cystic degeneration within the inflamed, thickened sinus lining. Regardless of the explanation, both lesions are termed *pseudocysts* because they have no epithelial lining.

Retention pseudocysts may be found in any of the paranasal sinuses at any time during the year, occurring most frequently around April and November. This timing suggests that the pseudocyst may be related to seasonal environmental changes.

Studies indicate that retention pseudocysts are more common in males and rarely cause symptoms. Because of an absence of signs and symptoms, the affected patient usually has no awareness of the lesion and, thus, the lesion is often noticed as an "incidental finding" on images made for other purposes. When a pseudocyst completely fills the maxillary sinus cavity, it may extrude through the ostium, causing nasal obstruction and postnasal discharge. Enlarged retention pseudocysts may rupture as a result of changes in pressure due to sneezing or nose blowing. Also, an expanded pseudocyst may herniate through the ostium into the nasal cavity, where it can rupture. The pseudocyst may be present on CT examination of the maxillary sinus one day, absent only a few days later, and then may reappear on a subsequent examination.

The maxillary sinus is the most common site of mucous retention pseudocysts, although they are occasionally found in the frontal or sphenoid sinuses. Mucous retention pseudocysts are not associated with extractions or periapical disease.

Radiographic Description

Retention pseudocysts appear as smooth, dome-shaped radiopaque masses with no osseous border. The base of the lesion may be narrow, although most have broad bases. Partial images of retention pseudocysts of the maxillary sinus may appear on the axial, coronal, and sagittal images of CBCT (Figure 4.28). Although pseudocysts

(a)

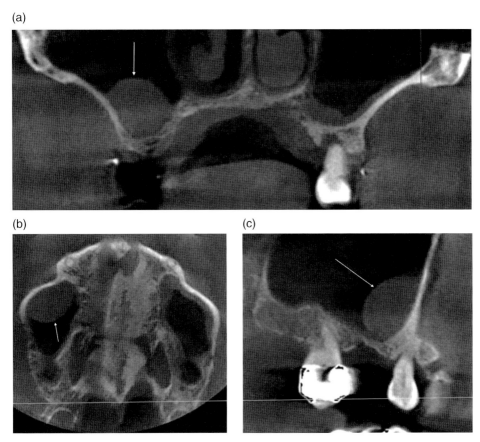

(b)   (c)

Figure 4.28. (a) Coronal view showing a radiopaque dome-shaped entity on the floor of the right maxillary sinus (white arrow) consistent with a retention pseudocyst and soft-tissue thickening of the left maxillary sinus consistent with sinusitis. (b) Axial view showing a radiopaque dome-shaped entity on the floor of the right maxillary sinus (white arrow) consistent with a retention pseudocyst and soft-tissue thickening of the left maxillary sinus consistent with sinusitis. (c) Sagittal view showing a radiopaque dome-shaped entity on the floor of the right maxillary sinus (white arrow) consistent with a retention pseudocyst.

may occur bilaterally, they usually develop unilaterally. Occasionally, multiple pseudocysts may form within one sinus. These pseudocysts usually project from the floor of the sinus; some may form on the lateral or medial walls of the antrum (Figure 4.29). The size of the mucous retention pseudocysts may vary from that of a fingertip to a size large enough to completely fill the sinus, causing the sinus to appear completely opacified (Figure 4.30). The roots of healthy teeth projecting over an area of an antral cavity occupied by a retention pseudocyst usually have intact lamina dura.

Imaging allows for differentiation between antral polyps of an infectious or allergic nature and antral retention pseudocysts in that they are more often seen in multiples. They are commonly associated with a thickened mucous membrane, a characteristic less frequently observed with retention pseudocysts.

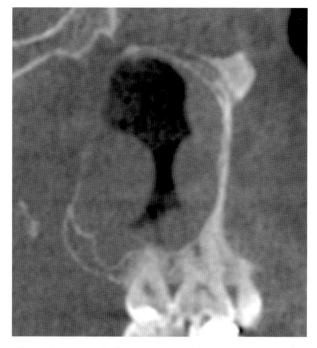

Figure 4.29.   Sagittal view showing multiple retention pseudocysts versus sinus polyposis.

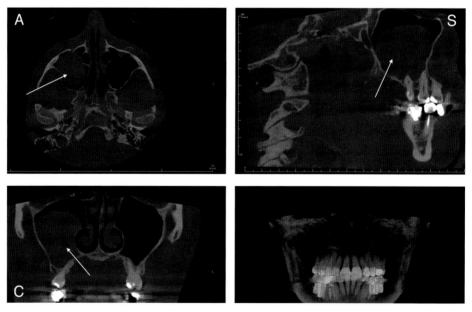

Figure 4.30.   Axial (A), coronal (C), and sagittal (S) views showing a large retention pseudocyst (white arrows) nearly filling the entire right maxillary sinus.

Differential Interpretation

Neoplasms may also mimic retention pseudocysts. If the neoplasms are benign and originate from outside the sinus, they are separated from the antrum of the sinus by a radiopaque border similar to that of odontogenic cysts. Malignant neoplasms may destroy the osseous border of the affected sinus, regardless of whether it arises from within the sinus or from the alveolar process. It is less likely that a neoplasm will appear as dome shaped as is characteristic of the mucous retention pseudocyst.

Treatment/Recommendations

Retention pseudocysts in the maxillary sinus usually require no treatment because they customarily resolve spontaneously without any residual effect on the antral mucosa.

Polyps

Definition/Clinical Characteristics

Polyp is the term used to describe irregular folds occurring in the thickened mucous membrane of a chronically inflamed sinus. Polyposis of the sinus mucosa may occur in an isolated area or in multiple sites throughout the sinus.

Radiographic Description

The internal structure of the polyp is homogeneous and more radiopaque than the surrounding sinus antrum's air-filled cavity. The radiopacity of the lesion is caused by the accumulation of fluid, thus leaving normal osseous landmarks visible through its image. Polyps may cause bony displacement and/or destruction. Polyps found in the ethmoid air cells may cause destruction of the medial wall of the orbit, the lamina papyracea of the ethmoid bone, causing a unilateral proptosis to develop. Polyps have no effect on the floor of the affected sinus, which remains intact.

Differential Interpretation

A polyp may be differentiated from a retention pseudocyst on a CT image by noting that a polyp usually occurs with a thickened mucous membrane lining because the polypoid mass is essentially an accentuation of the mucosal thickening. In the case of a mucous retention pseudocyst, an adjacent mucous membrane lining is not seen. If multiple mucous retention pseudocysts are seen within a sinus, sinus polyposis (Figures 4.29 and 4.31) should be part of the differential diagnosis. The radiographic image of the bone displacement or destruction associated with polyps may mimic a benign or malignant neoplasm.

Treatment/Recommendations

Because many sinus neoplasms are asymptomatic, examination of a paranasal sinus evidencing bony destruction associated with radiopacification should lead to biopsy.

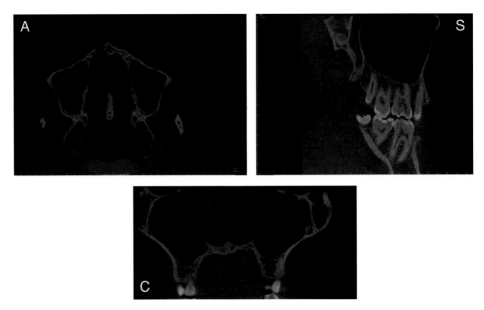

Figure 4.31.   Axial (A), coronal (C), and sagittal (S) views showing multiple nodular areas with soft-tissue thickening of the maxillary sinuses suggestive of sinus polyposis.

Empyema

Definition/Clinical Characteristics/Radiographic Description

An empyema is a pus-filled space that may be the result of blockage of the sinus ostium by a thickened, inflamed mucous membrane or another pathologic process, especially in cases where the maxillary sinus is involved. Empyema is most likely a variant of the mucocele or pyocele.

Antrolith

Definition/Clinical Characteristics

Antroliths occur within the maxillary sinuses and are the result of the deposition of mineral salts such as calcium phosphate, calcium carbonate, and magnesium around a nidus, which has been introduced into the sinus through either an extrinsic or intrinsic mechanism. Smaller antroliths are asymptomatic and are discovered as "incidental findings" on radiographic examination. If a small antrolith continues its growth, the patient may experience an associated sinusitis with bloody nasal discharge, a nasal obstruction, or facial pain.

Radiographic Description

Antroliths occur within the maxillary sinus superior to the floor of the maxillary antrum in axial, coronal, and sagittal CT. Antroliths are well defined and may have a smooth or irregular shape. The internal structure may vary in density from a slight radiopacity to extreme radiopacity. The internal density may be homogenous or heterogeneous. In some instances, layers of radiolucency and radiopacity are seen, appearing as laminations (Figures 4.32 and 4.33).

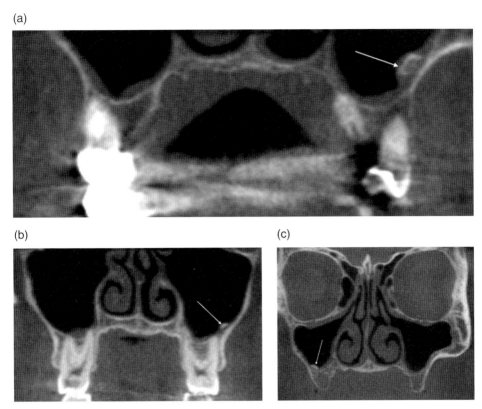

Figure 4.32. (a) Coronal view showing a calcified entity (white arrow) in the left maxillary sinus consistent with an antrolith. (b) Coronal view showing a calcified entity (white arrow) in the left maxillary sinus consistent with an antrolith. (c) Coronal view showing a calcified entity (white arrow) in the right maxillary sinus consistent with an antrolith.

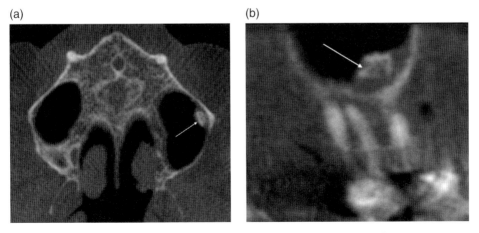

Figure 4.33. (a) Axial view showing a calcified entity (white arrow) in the left maxillary sinus consistent with an antrolith. (b) Sagittal view showing a calcified entity (white arrow) in the maxillary sinus consistent with an antrolith.

Differential Interpretation

Antroliths may be distinguished from root fragments in the sinus by inspection of the mass for the normal root anatomy, specifically the presence of a pulp canal.

Treatment/Recommendations

Referral to an ear, nose, and throat physician or primary care physician is recommended to determine if further treatment such as surgical removal is necessary.

Mucocele

Definition/Clinical Characteristics

A mucocele is an expanding, destructive lesion resulting from blockage of a sinus ostium. The blockage may be the result of intra-antral or intranasal inflammation, a polyp, or a neoplasm. Thus, the entire sinus becomes a cystlike lesion. Accumulated mucus fills the sinus cavity and increases the intra-antral pressure, which then results in a thinning, displacement, and, often, destruction of the sinus walls. If the mucocele becomes infected, it is called a pyocele or amucopyocele.

The effect of pressure from a mucocele in the maxillary sinus may be radiating pain produced in the region of the superior alveolar nerves. First, the patient may complain of a sensation of cheek fullness and swelling. This swelling may become apparent over the anteroinferior aspect of the antrum where the wall of the sinus is thin or destroyed. Inferior expansion of the lesion may cause loosening of posterior teeth. If the medial wall of the sinus is expanded, the lateral wall of the nasal cavity will deform, which may contribute to obstruction of the nasal airway. When expansion includes the orbit, diplopia or proptosis may occur.

Radiographic Description

With bony expansion comes a change in the shape of the sinus. Septa and the bony walls may be thinned and/or destroyed. When the mucocele is associated with the maxillary sinus antrum, teeth may be displaced or roots may be resorbed. In the frontal sinus, expansion causes smoothing of the usually scalloped border and, potentially, displacement of the intersinus septum. The orbit's supramedial border may be displaced or destroyed. In the ethmoid air cells, displacement of the lamina papyracea may occur, contributing to displacement of the orbital contents. In the sphenoid sinus, expansion occurs superiorly and may be suggestive of a pituitary neoplasm. About 90% of mucoceles occur in the ethmoidal (Figure 4.34) and frontal sinuses and are rare in the maxillary and sphenoid sinuses.

Differential Interpretation

While it may not be possible to distinguish a mucocele located in the maxillary antrum from a cyst or neoplasm, a suggestion that the lesion is associated with an occluded ostium increases the likelihood that the lesion is indeed a mucocele. Blockage of the ostium is usually the result of a prior surgical procedure, although a deviated nasal septum or polyp may be a factor. A large odontogenic cyst displacing the maxillary antral floor may mimic a mucocele. CT is the imaging method of choice for differentiating these entities.

(a)

(b)

(c)

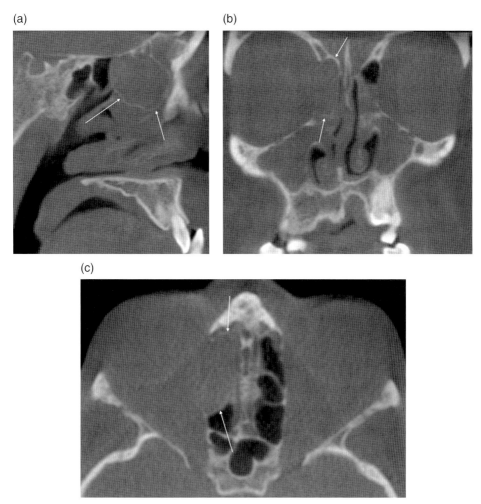

Figure 4.34. (a) Sagittal view showing a mucocele (white arrows) of the ethmoid air cells altering the shape the air cell borders. (b) Coronal view showing a mucocele (white arrows) of the right ethmoid air cells. (c) Axial view showing a mucocele (white arrows) of the right ethmoid air cells altering the shape of the air cell borders.

Treatment

Treatment of a mucocele is usually surgical, using a Caldwell–Luc procedure to allow excision of the lesion. The prognosis is excellent.

Postsurgical Changes of Paranasal Sinuses

Uncinectomy

Definition

One of the most accepted means of functionally enlarging the maxillary ostium is to perform an uncinectomy via the "swing door" technique. This initially removes the vertical process of the uncinate via backbiter inferiorly and sickle knife superiorly.

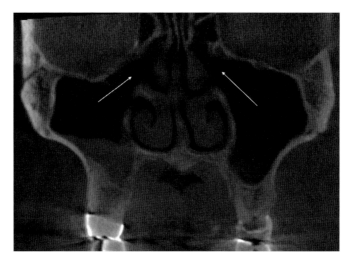

Figure 4.35.   Coronal view showing bilateral uncinectomy (white arrows) creating an enlarged drainage for the maxillary sinuses.

The uncinate is swung medially and then severed at its lateral attachment. This is followed by a submucosal removal of the horizontal process of the uncinate and subsequent trimming of the mucosa to fully visualize the maxillary ostium.

Controversy exists as to whether or not the maxillary ostium should be enlarged or not depending on the disease status of the maxillary sinus. However, the medical literature would support a wide antrostomy and complete clearance down to healthy mucosa if fungal mucin is present within the sinus.

Radiographic Description

In this circumstance, the ostium is enlarged superiorly to orbital floor and posteriorly to posterior fontanelle to allow wide access for clearance (Figure 4.35).

Caldwell–Luc Procedure

Definition/Radiographic Description

For persistent symptoms and disease in patients who have failed medical and functional endoscopic approaches, older techniques can be used to address the inflammation of the maxillary sinus, such as the Caldwell–Luc radical antrostomy. This surgery involves an incision in the upper gum, opening in the anterior wall of the antrum, and removal of the entire diseased maxillary sinus mucosa. Drainage is allowed into inferior or middle meatus by creating a large window in the lateral nasal wall.

References

Bent, J. P., Cuilty-Siller, C., Kuhn, F. A. (1994). The frontal cell as a cause of frontal sinus obstruction. *American Journal of Rhinology*, 7, 185–91.

Dolan, K. D. (1982). Paranasal sinus radiology, part 2A: ethmoidal sinuses. *Head and Neck*, July/August, 486.

Gotwald, T. F., Zinreich, S. J., Fishman, E. K. (2001). Three-dimensional volumetric display of the nasal ostiomeatal channels and paranasal sinuses. *Am J Rhinology*, January, 176, 241–5.

Huang, B. Y., Lloyd, K. M., DelGaudio, J. M., et al. (2009). Failed endoscopic sinus surgery: spectrum of CT findings in the frontal recess. *Radiographics*, **29**(1), 177–95.

Mallaya, S., and Lam, E. (Ed.). (2019) *White and Pharaoh's Oral Radiology: Principles and Interpretation*. Mosby.

Som, P. M., and Curtin, H. D. (2003). *Head and Neck Imaging*, Volumes 1 and 2. Mosby.

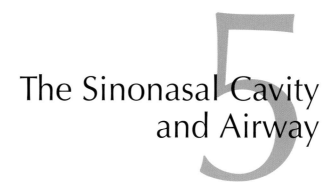

The Sinonasal Cavity and Airway

Gayle Tieszen Reardon

Introduction

This chapter covers the sinonasal cavity and airway. It is common for allergies and infectious diseases to affect not only the paranasal sinuses but also the nasal cavities. Therefore, the nasal cavity is a partner with the paranasal sinuses in terms of frequency for imaging indications. In addition to allergies and infectious diseases, facial fractures are common and may range from a broken nose to more complex fractures secondary to traumas. Also, there are disfiguring tumors of the sinonasal cavities that have poor prognoses and wreak facial carnage, thus contributing to their fearsome reputations.

Anatomy

Nose is the term generally used to describe the pyramid-shaped external soft tissue projecting ventral to the surface of the face. Nasal fossa, or nasal cavities, refer to the internal nasal airways.

Topographically, the nose is divided into subunits that have practical importance for reconstructive surgeons. The subunits consist of the nasal dorsum, the nasal sidewalls, the nasal tip and columella, the alar lobule, and the supraalar facets. The nasion is the junction of the root of the nose with the forehead. The lower or caudal free margin of the nose is formed by the alar rim, columella, and tip. Bilaterally, the lateral lower margin of the nose has a rounded expansile region referred to as the alar lobule and consists of skin and soft tissue posterior and inferior to the lateral crus of the lower lateral cartilage. The dorsum of the nose consists of the nasal bones' dorsal surfaces superiorly and the dorsal border of the quadrangular cartilage attaching to the upper lateral cartilages inferomedially. The junction of the alae with the face is known as the alar-facial junction.

Interpretation Basics of Cone Beam Computed Tomography, Second Edition.
Edited by Shawneen M. Gonzalez.
© 2021 John Wiley & Sons, Inc. Published 2021 by John Wiley & Sons, Inc.
Companion website: www.wiley.com/go/gonzalez/interpretation

Som and Curtin (2003) describe the journey of inspired air as it enters the nasal cavity in the following manner:

> Inspired air traverses the nasal valve. This is a circular area encompassed by the nasal septum, upper lateral cartilage, tip of the inferior turbinate, and floor of the nose. The total area encompassed by this valve provides the most important resistance to air flow in the nasal cavity. Of slightly lesser importance is the angle formed by the meeting of the quadrangular cartilage of the nasal septum and the inferior border of the upper lateral cartilages which is known as the nasal valve angle. Due to its mobile nature, it is a dynamic structure that narrows and widens with the phases of respiration. It is thus a critical factor in determining airflow through the nasal cavity.

The two sides of the nasal cavity are separated by the nasal septum. The septum supports the bony and cartilaginous vault and the tip of the nose. The main components of the nasal septum are the vomer, the perpendicular plate of the ethmoid, the quadrangular cartilage, the membranous septum, and the columella. The vomer may be bilaminar due to its embryologic origin; the vomer and the perpendicular plate of the ethmoid bone may become pneumatized.

The perpendicular plate of the ethmoid bone fuses with the cribriform plate superiorly. The vomer articulates superiorly with the perpendicular plate of the ethmoid and the crest of the sphenoid, anteriorly with the quadrangular cartilage, and inferiorly with the palatine bone and nasal crest of the maxilla. The thin groove of the quadrangular cartilage has a "tongue-in-groove" relationship with the vomer. The posterior border of the vomer is free and divides the posterior choanae.

The inferior turbinate (concha) is a separate bone of the skull. The inferior turbinate is larger than the other turbinates. The nasolacrimal duct drains tears into the inferior meatus. The superior and middle conchae are parts of the ethmoid bone. The middle meatus receives drainage from the frontal sinus (via the frontal recess), drains through the middle meatus, or infundibulum to middle meatus, to the nasal cavity, to the nasopharynx. The maxillary sinus (via the maxillary ostium) drains through the infundibulum, the middle meatus, the nasal cavity, and, finally, the nasopharynx. The anterior ethmoid air cells drain via the anterior ethmoid ostia into the nasal cavity. In the ethmoid bone, the uncinate process is a curved lamina that projects downward and backward from this part of the labyrinth. It forms a small part of the medial wall of the maxillary sinus and articulates with the ethmoid process of the inferior nasal concha (Figures 5.1–5.8).

Normal Anatomy of the Ostiomeatal Complex

See Chapter 4 for additional information.

Anatomical Variations of the Nasal Septum

The nasal septum is fundamental to the development of the nose and paranasal sinuses. Deviations of the nasal septum are usually congenital but may be due to previous experiences of trauma in some patients. Developmentally, there may be malalignment of the components of the nasal septum (the septal cartilage, perpendicular ethmoid bone, and vomer), which may cause deviation of the nasal septum,

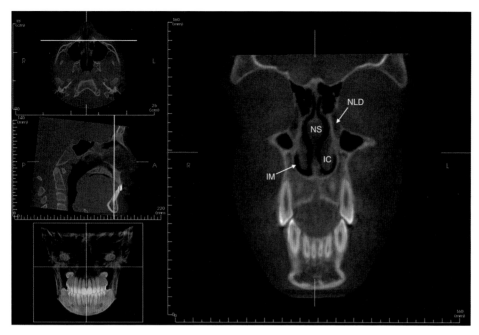

Figure 5.1. Coronal view showing the nasolacrimal duct (NLD), nasal septum (NS), inferior concha (IC), and inferior meatus (IM). Yellow line showing coronal plane on left views (axial and sagittal).

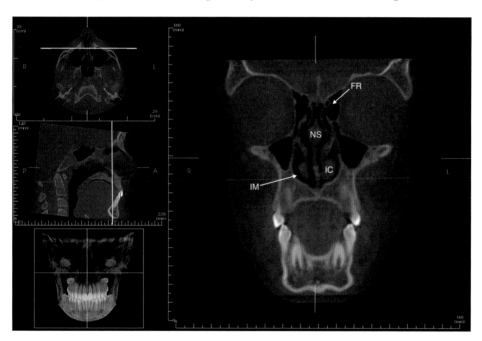

Figure 5.2. Coronal view showing the frontal recess (FR), nasal septum (NS), inferior concha (IC), and inferior meatus (IM). Yellow line showing coronal plane on left views (axial and sagittal).

deformities of the tongue-in-groove relationship of the cartilage and vomer, or a septal bony spur. About one-third of septal deviations are asymptomatic; however, more severe chondrovomer articulation problems may contribute to sinusitis symptoms. Obstruction, secondary inflammation, and infection of the middle meatus have been observed secondary to severe nasal septal deviations (Figures 5.9 and 5.10).

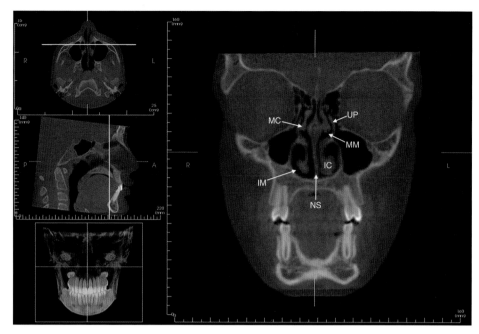

Figure 5.3.   Coronal view showing the uncinate process (UP), middle meatus (MM), inferior concha (IC), nasal septum (NS), inferior meatus (IM), and middle concha (MC). Yellow line showing coronal plane on left views (axial and sagittal).

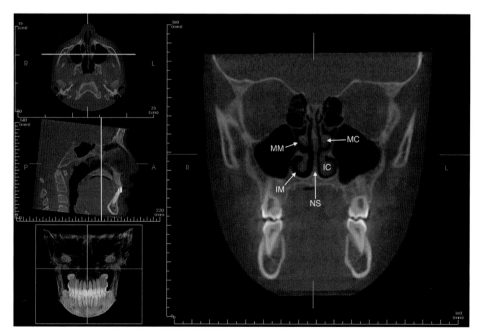

Figure 5.4.   Coronal view showing the middle concha (MC), middle meatus (MM), inferior concha (IC), inferior meatus (IM), and nasal septum (NS). Yellow line showing coronal plane on left views (axial and sagittal).

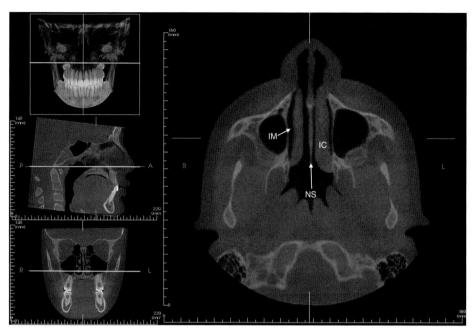

Figure 5.5. Axial view showing the inferior meatus (IM), inferior concha (IC), and nasal septum (NS). Yellow line showing axial plane on left views (3D reconstruction, sagittal, and coronal).

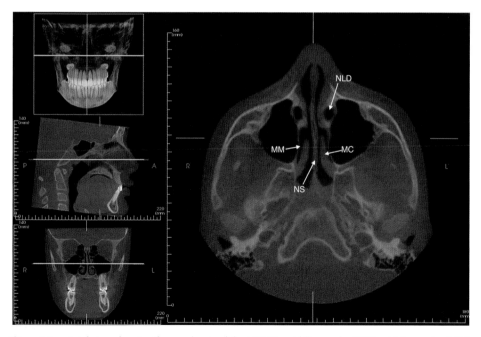

Figure 5.6. Axial view showing the nasolacrimal duct (NLD), middle concha (MC), middle meatus (MM), and nasal septum (NS). Yellow line showing axial plane on left views (3D reconstruction, sagittal, and coronal).

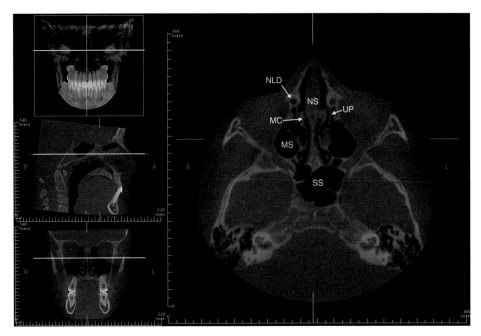

Figure 5.7. Axial view showing the nasolacrimal duct (NLD), nasal septum (NS), middle concha (MC), uncinate process (UP), maxillary sinuses (MS), and sphenoid sinuses (SS). Yellow line showing axial plane on left views (3D reconstruction, sagittal, and coronal).

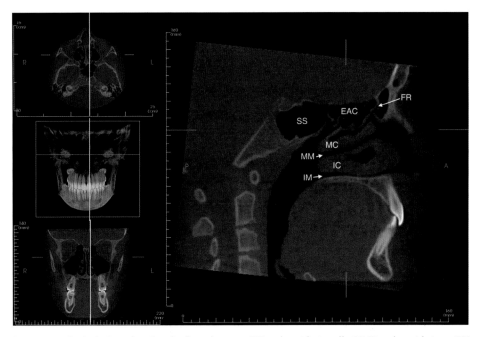

Figure 5.8. Sagittal view showing the frontal recess (FR), ethmoid air cells (EAC), sphenoid sinus (SS), middle concha (MC), middle meatus (MM), inferior concha (IC), and inferior meatus (IM). Yellow line showing sagittal plane on left views (axial, 3D reconstruction, and coronal).

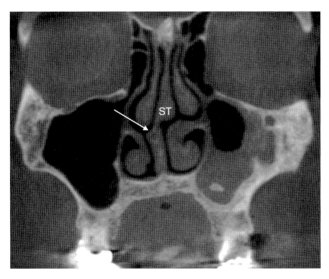

Figure 5.9. Coronal view showing nasal septum deviation to the right (white arrow) with enlargement of the septal cartilage [septal tubercle (ST)].

(a) (b)

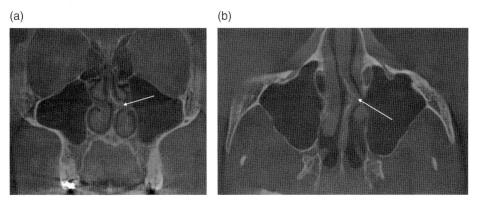

Figure 5.10. (a) Coronal view showing left-sided bony spur formation at the level of the middle meatus (white arrow). (b) Axial view showing left-sided bony spur formation (white arrow).

Anatomical Variations of the Middle Turbinate

There are several variations of the middle turbinate including paradoxic curvature, concha bullosa, lamellar concha, medial/lateral displacement, L-shaped lateral branding, and sagittal transverse clefts. The first three, which are more common, are described in detail below.

Paradoxic Curvature

Normally the curvature of the middle turbinate is directed laterally, toward the lateral sinus wall. When paradoxically curved, the curvature is directed medially toward the nasal septum. The inferior edge of the middle turbinate may take on excessive curvature, which may then narrow or obstruct the nasal cavity, infundibulum, or middle meatus. Because of the potential narrowing and/or obstruction associated with paradoxic curvature, it is considered a contributing factor to sinusitis by authors Som and Curtin (2003) (Figure 5.11).

Concha Bullosa

A concha bullosa is an aerated turbinate; the turbinate most often associated with concha bullosa is the middle turbinate (Figures 5.12–5.14). Concha bullosa may be either unilateral or bilateral; however, it is more frequently bilateral in its presentation. Less frequently, aeration of the superior turbinate may occur; an aerated inferior turbinate is uncommon. Classifications of concha bullosa are divided according to degree of turbinate pneumatization. When the pneumatization involves the bulbous segment of the middle turbinate, the term *concha bullosa* applies. If the pneumatization is limited to the attachment portion of the middle turbinate and does not extend

(a)   (b)

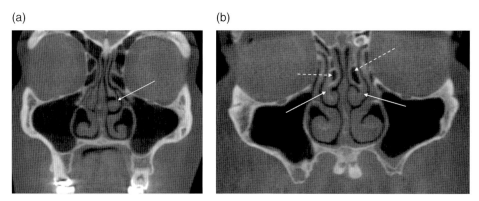

Figure 5.11.   (a) Coronal view showing paradoxical curvature of the left middle concha (white arrow). (b) Coronal view showing bilateral paradoxical curvature of the middle conchae (white arrows) with bilateral lamellar concha at the attachment of middle conchae (white dashed arrows).

(a)   (b)

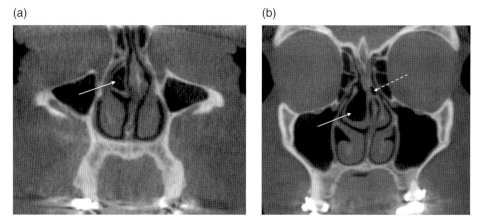

Figure 5.12.   (a) Coronal view showing an aerated concha consistent with concha bullosa of the right middle concha (white arrow). (b) Coronal view showing an aerated concha consistent with concha bullosa (white arrow) of the right middle concha and lamellar concha (white dashed arrow) of the left middle concha.

(a)

(b)

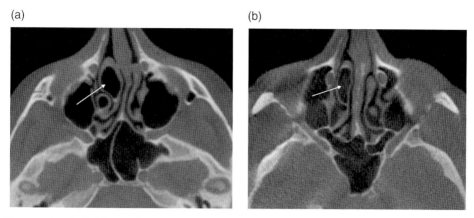

Figure 5.13. (a) Axial view showing an aerated concha consistent with concha bullosa of the right middle concha (white arrow). (b) Axial view showing an aerated concha consistent with concha bullosa of the right middle concha (white arrow).

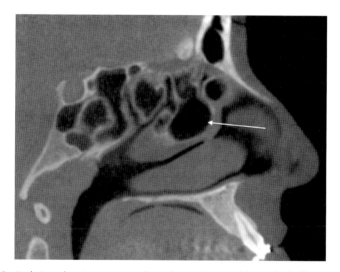

Figure 5.14. Sagittal view showing an aerated concha consistent with concha bullosa (white arrow).

into the bulbous segment, it is called lamellar concha. A concha bullosa of the middle turbinate may cause enlargement of the turbinate such that the middle meatus or infundibulum are obstructed, thus associating concha bullosa with a higher prevalence of ipsilateral sinus disease.

Lamellar Concha

Only the attachment portion of the middle turbinate is pneumatized, and the pneumatization does not extend into the bulbous segment (Figures 5.11b, 5.12b, and 5.15).

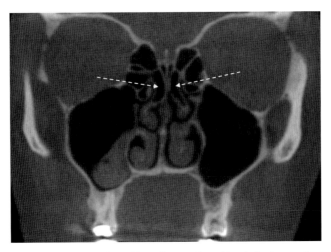

Figure 5.15.   Coronal view showing bilateral lamellar concha (white dashed arrows).

Anatomy of the Uncinate Process

Attachment

Normally, the upper tip of the uncinate process attaches to the lateral nasal wall where the agger nasi cells are commonly located. Anatomic variations of the uncinate attachment include attachment to the lamina papyracea, the lateral surface of the middle turbinate, or the fovea ethmoidalis in the floor of the anterior cranial fossa. Sometimes the free edge of the uncinate process may adhere to the orbital floor or the inferior aspect of the lamina papyracea, a condition known as an atelectatic uncinate process; this is associated with a hypoplastic, and often opacified, ipsilateral maxillary sinus secondary to closure of the infundibulum. Yet another variant of the uncinate process configuration is its extension superiorly to the roof of the anterior ethmoid sinus, causing the superior infundibulum to end as a "blind pouch." This continuation of the uncinate is referred to as lamina terminalis. In these causes, the infundibulum drains via the posterior aspect of the middle meatus.

The uncinate process may also become pneumatized, a condition referred to as uncinate bulla (Figures 5.16 and 5.17). Uncinate bulla is considered a predisposing factor for impaired sinus ventilation in the anterior ethmoid, frontal recess, and infundibular regions. Functionally, the pneumatized uncinate process resembles concha bullosa and is believed to be an extension of the agger nasi cell within the anterosuperior portion of the uncinate process.

Deviation

The uncinate process is one of the crucial bony structures of the wall of the lateral nasal cavity. The uncinate process together with the ethmoid bulla form the boundaries of the hiatus semilunaris and ethmoid infundibulum, the structures through which the frontal and maxillary sinuses drain. It is the free edge of the uncinate process that may vary in configuration. Medial and lateral deviation of uncinate process may cause narrowing or obstruction of the middle meatus, the hiatus semilunaris, and infundibulum.

(a)   (b)

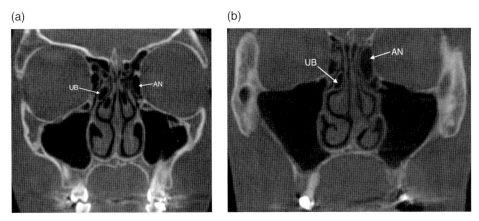

Figure 5.16. (a) Coronal view showing an aerated right uncinate process consistent with uncinate bulla (UB) and left agger nasi cells (AN). (b) Coronal view showing an aerated right uncinate process consistent with uncinate bulla (UB) and left agger nasi cells (AN).

(a)   (b)

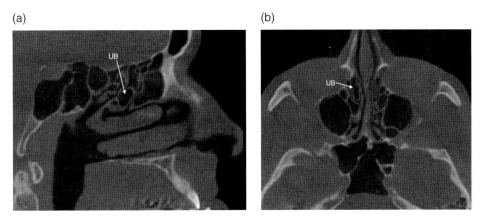

Figure 5.17. (a) Sagittal view showing an aerated uncinate process consistent with uncinate bulla (UB). (b) Axial view showing an aerated right uncinate process consistent with uncinate bulla (UB).

Anatomy of the Frontal Recess

The frontal recess is an hourglass-like narrowing between the frontal sinus and the anterior middle meatus through which the frontal sinus drains. It is not a tubular structure, as "nasofrontal duct" might imply, thus the use of the term *frontal recess*. The frontal recesses are the narrowest anterior air channel and common site of inflammation resulting in loss of ventilation and mucociliary clearance of the frontal sinus (Figures 5.2 and 5.8).

The boundaries of the frontal recess are agger nasi cells anteriorly and the ethmoid bulla, its associated bulla lamella, and the suprabullar cell (if present) posteriorly. The lateral border is the lamina papyracea. The medial border is the most anterior and superior portion of the middle turbinate.

In approximately 40% of cases, secretions from the frontal recess drain into the ethmoid infundibulum and subsequently into the middle meatus through the hiatus semilunaris. In the remaining cases, the frontal recess drains directly into the middle meatus.

The frontal recess may be pneumatized by various anterior ethmoid cells, which are collectively known as frontal recess cells. These cells are normal anatomic variations that are present in some combination in most individuals. The clinical relevance of frontal recess cells lies in their potential for causing frontal sinusitis by obstructing frontal sinus outflow at the level of the frontal recess. Any endoscopic surgical procedure aimed at clearing frontal recess obstruction must address these variant cells; failure to do so may result in surgical failure. For this reason, the radiologist's report must accurately characterize any frontal recess cells present by using standard accepted nomenclature.

The frontal recess cells include agger nasi cells, frontal cells (type 1, 2, 3, and 4), supraorbital ethmoid cells, frontal bullar cells, suprabullar cells, and interfrontal sinus septal cells. The frontal cells along with the agger nasi cells constitute the anterior group of frontal recess cells

The supraorbital ethmoid cells, frontal bullar cells, and suprabullar cells make up the posterior group of frontal recess cells. All of the cells in this group are located along the posterior wall of the frontal recess and are bordered posteriorly or superiorly by the anterior skull base.

Agger Nasi Cell

Agger nasi is a Latin term meaning "nasal mound." The agger nasi appears as an eminence located on the lateral nasal wall at the leading edge of the middle turbinate; it represents the intranasal portion of the frontal process of the maxilla. The agger nasi serves as the anterior limit of the frontal recess. Pneumatization of the agger nasi (resulting in the agger nasi cell) occurs in 78% to 98.5% of individuals. When present, agger nasi cells are considered the most anterior of all ethmoid cells and can pneumatize posteriorly to narrow the frontal recess (Figures 5.16, 5.18 and 5.19).

Frontal Cells

Frontal cells, along with the agger nasi cell, constitute the anterior group of frontal recess cells. Frontal cells are present on computed tomography (CT) in 20% to 33% of patients. The anterior boundaries of these cells are made up of the anterior wall of the frontal recess or the frontal sinus; these cells do not extend posteriorly to abut

(a)   (b)

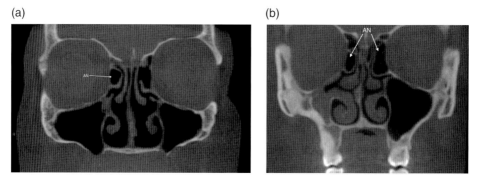

Figure 5.18.   (a) Coronal view showing right agger nasi cell (AN) directly medial to the orbital cavity. (b) Coronal view showing bilateral agger nasi cells (AN) directly medial to the orbital cavity.

the skull base. There are four types of frontal cells described under the system known as the Kuhn classification.

Type 1 Frontal Cells

Seen in up to 37% of frontal recesses, type 1 cells are defined as single anterior ethmoid cells within the frontal recess sitting above the agger nasi cell. These cells do not extend into the frontal sinus (Figure 5.19).

Type 2 Frontal Cells

Seen in up to 19% of frontal recesses, type 2 cells are defined as a tier of two or more anterior ethmoid cells sitting above the agger nasi cell (Figure 5.20).

Type 3 Frontal Cells

Seen in approximately 7% of frontal recesses. The type 3 cells are a single large cell above the agger nasi cell that extends into the frontal sinus.

(a) (b)

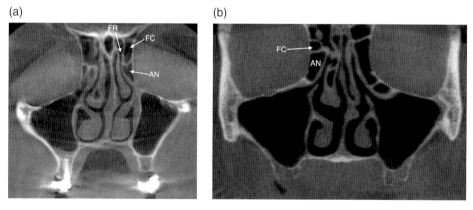

Figure 5.19. (a) Coronal view showing type 1 frontal cell (FC) directly superior to agger nasi cell (AN) and lateral to the frontal recess (FR). (b) Coronal view showing type 1 frontal cell (FC) directly medial to the right orbital cavity and superior to an agger nasi cell (AN).

(a) (b)

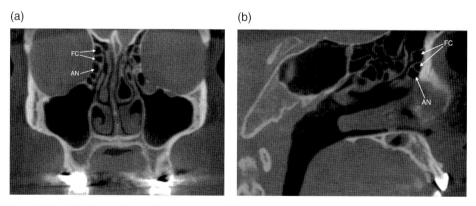

Figure 5.20. (a) Coronal view showing type 2 frontal cells (FC) superior to an agger nasi cell (AN). (b) Sagittal view showing type 2 frontal cells (FC) superior to an agger nasi cell (AN).

Type 4 Frontal Cells

Type 4 frontal cells account for 2.4% of all frontal recesses. Type 4 frontal cells are unique among the frontal cells in that they do not directly touch the agger nasi cell. They are defined as an isolated air cell located within the frontal sinus. It is bordered anteriorly by the anterior frontal sinus table, with their posterior walls representing free partitions in the frontal sinus. Recognition of type 4 cells often requires both coronal and sagittal CT reformation. On sagittal images, these cells have been described as having the appearance of a "balloon on a string," with the cell itself representing the balloon and the narrow outflow tract of the cell representing the string. Most often, type 4 cells have no identifiable connection to the frontal recess on imaging. In patients with frontal sinus disease, an isolated aerated cell abutting the anterior sinus wall in an otherwise opacified frontal sinus (the "cell within a cell") usually represents a type 4 frontal cell. It has been observed that frontal mucosal thickening is more prevalent in patients with type 3 and type 4 frontal cells than in those without frontal cells.

Supraorbital Ethmoid Cells

The supraorbital ethmoid cells are anterior ethmoid air cells that extend superiorly and laterally over the orbit from the frontal recess. These cells represent pneumatization of the orbital plate of the frontal bone posterior to the frontal recess and the frontal sinus. Identification of these cells at CT requires review of both axial and coronal images (Figure 5.21). They typically drain into the lateral aspect of the frontal recess. Up to 15% of adults may have one or more supraorbital ethmoid cells, with approximately 5% of frontal sinuses having multiple supraorbital cells. Supraorbital ethmoid cells can obstruct frontal sinus drainage. Pre-operative identification is essential because these cells can be readily mistaken for the frontal ostium during endoscopic dissection.

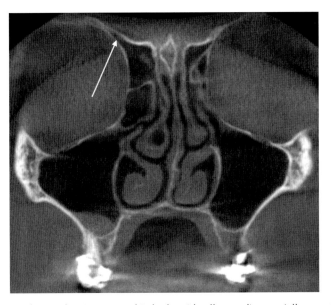

Figure 5.21.   Coronal view showing supraorbital ethmoid cell extending partially superior to the right orbit (white arrow).

Frontal Bullar Cells

This presents as a pneumatization of the anterior skull base in the posterior frontal recess with extension into the true frontal sinus. These cells lie above the ethmoid bulla and, when present, define a portion of the posterior boundary of the frontal recess and frontal sinus.

Suprabullar Cells

Suprabullar cells are nearly identical to frontal bullar cells, with the only distinguishing feature being that suprabullar cells lie entirely below the level of the frontal sinus ostium and do not extend into the frontal sinus. They sit above the ethmoid bulla and form a portion of the posterior wall of the frontal recess. They are best demonstrated on sagittal CT images. The suprabullar cell is bordered superiorly by the skull base; however, unlike a frontal bullar cell, the suprabullar cell does not extend above the level of the frontal ostium into the frontal sinus. During endoscopic frontal sinusotomy, both suprabullar and frontal bullar cells can be mistaken for the skull base; failure to recognize their presence pre-operatively can result in incomplete surgical dissection.

Interfrontal Sinus Septal Cells

The interfrontal sinus septal cell represents pneumatization of the interfrontal sinus septum. When extensive, such pneumatization can extend into the crista galli. These cells drain into the medial frontal recess and can impinge on the frontal sinus. Axial and coronal are the best planes for demonstrating these cells.

Surgical Variations

Frontal Sinuses

Endoscopic Frontal Recess Approach (Draf Type I Procedure)

This surgery consists of removal of obstructing structures, including anterosuperior ethmoid cells (agger nasi cell and any obstructing frontal recess cells) and the uncinate process. The dissection does not extend above the frontal ostium, hence the nasofrontal beak remains (best seen on the sagittal image).

Extended Frontal Sinusotomy (Draf Type II Procedure)

This procedure can be difficult to distinguish from the less-invasive endoscopic frontal recess approach (Draf type I surgery) at postoperative CT. Unlike the Draf type I procedure, Draf type II surgery includes resection of the frontal sinus floor and may extend into the frontal sinus, resulting in a less pronounced or absent nasofrontal beak on sagittal images.

Modified Lothrop Procedure (Draf Type III Procedure)

This procedure consists of contiguous bilateral enlargement of the frontal outflow tract, a result achieved by removal of the frontal sinus floors and adjacent parts of

(a)   (b)

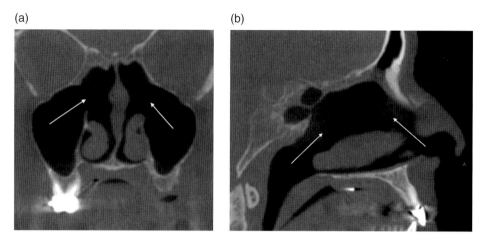

Figure 5.22.   (a) Coronal view showing Draf type III surgery (white arrows). (b) Sagittal view showing Draf type III surgery (white arrows).

the inferior interfrontal sinus septum, superior nasal septum, and anterior middle turbinates (Figure 5.22).

FESS Failure in Frontal Recess

Most cases of recurrent frontal sinusitis after functional endoscopic sinus surgery (FESS) can be attributed to stenosis of the frontal recess caused by:

1. Inadequate removal of the agger nasi and frontal recess cells.
2. A retained superior portion of the uncinate process.
3. Lateralization of the middle turbinate.
4. Osteoneogenesis secondary to chronic inflammation or mucosal stripping.
5. Scarring or inflammatory mucosal thickening.
6. Recurrent polyposis.

Residual Frontal Recess Cells

Postoperative coronal and sagittal CT images obtained through the left frontal recess show complete opacification of the frontal sinus and frontal recess. There are remnant opacified frontal recess cells, including an agger nasi cell and a tier of type 2 frontal cells, which narrow the frontal ostium and frontal recess.

Effect of the Superior Attachment of the Uncinate Process on Frontal Recess Drainage

The uncinate process has attached to the lamina papyracea. As a result, the ethmoid infundibulum terminates in a "blind recess" known as the recessus terminalis. In this case, frontal recess drainage passes directly into the middle meatus.

Coronal CT image shows the uncinate process attached to the skull base at the junction of the cribriform plate and lateral lamella. Therefore, frontal recess drainage is directed into the ethmoid infundibulum. In patients who have not undergone surgery, one of the most common causes of obstruction at the level of the frontal recess is a medially displaced uncinate process. This occurs when disease in the recessus terminalis displaces the uncinate process medially so that it lies close to or even against the middle turbinate. Occasionally, the uncinate process and middle turbinate may become fused. It is not uncommon for surgeons to ignore the superior attachment of the uncinate process. Not surprisingly, if a medialized uncinate process is left behind during FESS, then the frontal recess will have a tendency to restenose postoperatively.

Retained Uncinate Process

The uncinate process is attached to the lamina papyracea and forms a recessus terminalis, which is opacified. The frontal recess is opacified at the level of the recessus terminalis. The medialized left middle turbinate may adhere to the nasal septum; this appearance is a normal and often expected postsurgical finding.

Lateralized Middle Turbinate Remnant

In patients who have undergone middle turbinate manipulations, including partial middle turbinate resection, the amputated anterior stump may lateralize and obstruct the frontal recess. It has been suggested that recurrent frontal sinusitis occurs significantly more often in patients who have undergone partial middle turbinate resection than in surgically treated patients with intact middle turbinates; recent studies have disputed this claim.

Inflammatory Diseases

CT of the paranasal sinuses should not be performed until 4–6 weeks after initiation of medical therapy, and scanning should be delayed in patients with acute upper respiratory infections. Review of both sagittal and coronal reformatted images together significantly improves the practitioner's ability to identify and measure the frontal recess and is critical in assessment of obstructing anterior ethmoid cells. Helical scanning with a maximum section thickness of no greater than 1 mm is recommended.

Sinusitis

Sinusitis accounts for approximately 11.6 million office-based outpatient visits annually. In a significant proportion of patients with sinusitis, medical management alone is insufficient, necessitating surgical management. FESS has become the treatment of choice for patients with medically refractory rhinosinusitis. FESS is performed more than 200,000 times per year in the United States. FESS has a published success rate of 76% to 98%. Up to 23% of patients require revision surgery. In patients presenting with sinusitis after FESS, the frontal sinus outflow tract is the region where disease recurrence is most likely to occur. In addition, most medically refractory disease of the frontal sinuses can be attributed to obstruction at the level of the frontal recess. The frontal recess is a notoriously difficult area to treat with endoscopy owing to its anterior location and its tight confines between the orbit and anterior skull base. Furthermore, the frontal recess has a significant predilection for stenosis after FESS. Evaluation of patients in whom FESS has failed typically includes

CT of the paranasal sinuses to identify the potential causes of sinus outflow tract stenosis. Practitioners need to be familiar with the complex anatomy of the frontal recess and the processes that may contribute to surgical failure in order to generate accurate and meaningful reports for the referring rhinologists (see Chapter 4 for more information on sinusitis).

Osteoneogenesis

Among the primary objectives of FESS is preservation of normal mucociliary function. Failure to preserve the normal mucosa will tend to result in scarring and osteoneogenesis. Osteoneogenesis, also referred to as osteitis or hyperostosis, refers to bone remodeling and new bone formation caused by chronic inflammation. Sinus CT demonstrates osteoneogenesis in 36% to 64% of patients with chronic rhinosinusitis, and the presence of hyperostosis at pre-operative CT has been shown to be a predictor of poorer surgical outcome after FESS. The relatively high prevalence of osteoneogenesis in postoperative patients is believed to be related to a combination of surgical mucosal trauma, persistent inflammation, and chronic refractory infection. As for the reason why the presence of osteoneogenesis may contribute to surgical failure, it has been suggested that osteitic bone remnants serve as an inflammatory nidus, inducing overlying mucosal edema and hypertrophy, which in turn may contribute to frontal recess stenosis. In normal individuals, the bony septa of the ethmoid sinuses have an average thickness of approximately 0.5 mm, with the upper limit of normal being about 1 mm. In addition, on axial images the middle turbinate measures, on average, 1.5 mm at its midpoint in thickness. The normal upper limit of the middle turbinate measures 2.5 mm. When seen on CT, osteoneogenesis appears as thickening of the ethmoid septa or sinus walls and is often accompanied by scarring or mucosal edema. There is associated mucosal thickening, which may represent inflamed edematous mucosa, scar tissue, or secretions, causing sinus opacification.

Scarring and Inflammatory Mucosal Thickening

Scarring and inflammatory mucosal thickening in the frontal recess are extremely common after FESS, even in asymptomatic patients not requiring revision surgery. Although mucosal disease probably plays a role in most cases of recurrent frontal sinusitis after FESS, its presence at CT or endoscopy does not necessarily correlate with the presence of symptoms after surgery. Chronic sinus disease may be underdiagnosed with CT, as mucosal disease may be endoscopically visible even when it is not seen at CT. It is impossible to differentiate scarring from inflamed edematous mucosa at CT because both appear as mucosal thickening, and they should be reported as such. Within the paranasal sinuses, mucosal thickness up to 3 mm may be normal. In evaluation of the frontal recess, it is generally sufficient to report the presence or absence of mucosal thickening and, when mucosal thickening is present, a representative measurement of the degree of mucosal thickness.

Recurrent Polyposis

Sinonasal polyps are among the most frequent complications of sinusitis and among the most common findings in patients undergoing sinus surgery. They are formed by expansion of fluid in the deep lamina propria of the sinonasal Schneiderian mucosa and are the most common expansile lesions in the nasal cavity. Polyps have been associated with multiple causes including infectious rhinosinusitis, cystic fibrosis, aspirin intolerance, and allergic fungal sinusitis. Sinonasal polyposis is considered a predictor of poorer surgical outcome (surgical failure rates of 75% have been reported in patients with extensive sinonasal polyposis before surgery). Recurrent polyposis is seen in 29.9% to 40% of patients undergoing revision FESS. On CT images, polyps are usually homogeneous soft-tissue masses with smooth convex borders and may be single or multiple. As they enlarge, they may fill a sinus and go on to remodel or even destroy adjacent bony structures. Postoperative coronal and sagittal CT images show opacification of the frontal sinuses and polypoid soft tissue completely opacifying the frontal recess, findings consistent with recurrent polyposis.

Other Causes of Frontal Recess Obstruction

- Previously undetected mucoceles
- Polyps
- Mucous retention cyst
- Neoplasms
- Fibro-osseous lesions

Conclusions

CT is an invaluable adjunct to diagnostic nasal endoscopy in identifying various causes of frontal recess obstruction after FESS. Proper interpretation of CT scans obtained in patients being considered for frontal recess revision surgery requires a clear understanding of frontal recess anatomy, which in turn requires reviewing images in axial, coronal, and sagittal planes. In addition, a working knowledge of the most common causes of surgical failure in the frontal recess will ensure that these entities are not overlooked during revision surgery. Recognition and effective communication of the presence of these findings should lead to better patient care and may reduce the likelihood of additional surgical failures.

The Pharynx

The pharynx extends behind the oral cavity from the skull base to the level of the caudal cricoid cartilage. The pharynx is a mucosa-lined musculomembranous tube, which has historically been subdivided into three sections, the nasopharynx extending from the skull base to the level of the hard palate, the oropharynx extending from the level of the hard palate to the level of the hyoid bone, and the hypopharynx extending from the level of the hyoid bone to the caudal cricoid cartilage.

The Nasopharynx

The nasopharynx is a stratified squamous and columnar epithelium-lined cavity situated at the superior-most aspect of the aerodigestive tract. It measures about 2 cm in diameter anteroposteriorly and 4 cm in length. The nasopharynx communicates anteriorly with the nasal cavity and inferiorly with the oropharyngeal cavity. It is limited superiorly by the base of the skull, posteriorly by the prevertebral musculature of C1 and C2, and laterally by the pharyngeal constrictors and deep soft-tissue planes of the parapharyngeal space and infratemporal fossa. The inferior margin of the nasopharynx is the level of the hard palate and Passavant's muscle, which opposes the soft palate when elevated. It is Passavant's ridge that meets the elevated soft palate to close off the nasopharynx during swallowing. Overlying the nasopharyngeal structures is the pharyngobasilar fascia, which attaches to the base of the skull superiorly and the medial pterygoid plate anteriorly but has a free inferior margin. Patency of the nasopharynx is retained by the pharyngobasilar fascia. The visceral fascia and pharyngeal constrictor muscles form the lateral soft tissue borders supported by a bony framework composed of the maxilla anteriorly, the mandible laterally, and the base of the skull and vertebral bodies posteriorly. The visceral fascia surrounds the nasopharyngeal mucosa and constrictor muscles separating the nasopharynx from the deep fascial spaces and is thought to be a barrier to the spread of infection and malignancy.

The superior border of the nasopharynx consists of part of the vomer and the body of the sphenoid bone. If not surgically removed or atrophied, adenoidal tissues are located in the midline of the roof of the nasopharynx. The lateral bony border of the nasopharynx is the medial plate of the pterygoid process of the sphenoid bone with the medial pterygoid muscle attaching on the medial surface of the lateral plate and the pterygoid fossa. The anterior part of the nasopharynx is in direct communication with the nasal cavity by way of the posterior nasal choanae. It communicates with the middle ear cavity via the Eustachian tubes, which gain access to the nasopharynx through the sinus of Morgagni, a defect in the anterior portion of the pharyngobasilar fascia, which is superior to the pharyngeal constrictor muscle and along the superior posterior border of the medial pterygoid plate. The sinus of Morgagni is also a route of entry into the pharynx for the levatorvelli palatine muscle; it is this pathway that may provide access to the parapharyngeal region and central skull base for advanced nasopharyngeal cancer spread. The openings of the Eustachian tubes are located about 1 cm posteroinferiorly to the inferior turbinate, which predisposes the Eustachian tubes to obstruction by nasopharyngeal masses. Such obstructions may result in serous otitis in 50% of patients with history of nasopharyngeal masses.

Just posterosuperiorly to the torus tubarius is the fossa of Rosenmuller, a mucosa-lined recess at the most laterosuperior aspect of the nasopharynx. The fossa of Rosenmuller is lateral to flexor muscles of the neck, longus capitis, and colli and is a common origination site for nasopharyngeal cancers.

It is not uncommon for children to present with prominent adenoids, which reach their maximal size around 5 years of age. Involution of the adenoids begins around the time of puberty, with the majority of adenoidal tissue being absent by 30 years of age. Normal adenoidal tissue is seen in adults in their 30s, 40s, and 50s; however, it is unusual for the adenoidal mass to extend up to the posterior margin of the medial pterygoid plate. The presence of such a mass in an older patient should be evaluated by a physician.

Anatomy

The size of the nasopharynx is approximately 2 cm (anterior to posterior) and 4 cm (superior to inferior). The boundaries are the nasal cavity communication via posterior nasal choanae and nasal septum anteriorly and the opening of the Eustachian tube (torus tubarius and fossa of Rosenmuller) posteriorly. The superior boundary is the base of the skull (C1 and C2). The inferior boundary is the soft palate and Passavant's ridge. The lateral boundaries are the superior constrictor muscles/visceral fascia.

The Eustachian tube is the most anterior of nasopharynx landmarks along the posterolateral wall of the nasopharynx, anterior to torus tubarius. It crosses superior constrictor muscle to reach the nasopharynx from the middle ear cavity. The torus tubarius is a prominent cartilaginous structure. The anterior forms the posterior lip of the Eustachian tube orifice. The lateral wall is formed by the fossa of Rosenmuller and the Eustachian tube opening. The inferior aspect is formed by the soft palate. The fossa of Rosenmuller is the nasopharynx extension posterosuperior to the middle end of the Eustachian tube just posterior and superior to torus tubarius. It may be up to 1.5 cm deep in an adult. Cranial nerve V_3 lies anteriolateral to apex of fossa within parapharyngeal space. The most common site of origin of nasopharyngeal cancers are type I—keratinizing squamous cell carcinoma; type II—nonkeratinizing epidermoid carcinoma; and type III—undifferentiated carcinoma. In ancient Greece, ancient Rome, and during the Middle Ages, the posterior opening of the nasal passage (Greek *choane* = funnel) was known as an anatomical structure.

Incidental Findings

Adenoidal Hyperplasia

Definition/Clinical Characteristics/Radiographic Description

Adenoidal hyperplasia is a common incidental finding in younger individuals. It is categorized by the amount of hyperplasia encroaching into the airway in thirds. Mild adenoidal hyperplasia is one-third encroachment of the airway (Figure 5.23). Moderate adenoidal hyperplasia is two-thirds encroachment of the airway (Figure 5.24). Marked adenoidal hyperplasia is greater than two-thirds encroachment of the airway (Figure 5.25).

Differential Interpretation/Treatment

In an older patient, adenoidal hyperplasia may indicate a possible tumor. No treatment is necessary as this is an incidental finding; however, if the patient is having breathing issues referral may be recommended.

The Oropharynx

The region inferior to the nasopharynx is divided into two major components: the oropharynx and the oral cavity. The oral cavity is inferior to the nasal fossa and the bilateral maxillary sinuses. The oropharynx is the area directly inferior to the nasopharynx and posterior to the oral cavity with its superior border formed by the soft

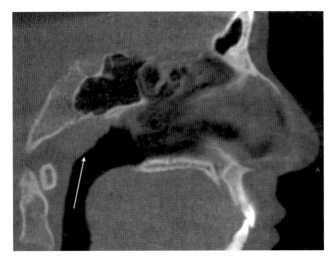

Figure 5.23.   Sagittal view on midline showing mild adenoidal hyperplasia (white arrow).

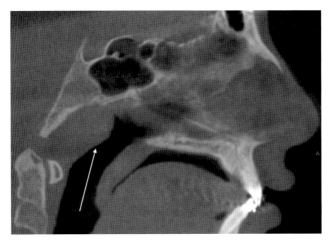

Figure 5.24.   Sagittal view on midline showing moderate adenoidal hyperplasia (white arrow).

(a)   (b)

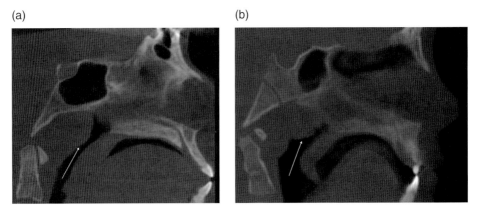

Figure 5.25.   (a) Sagittal view on midline showing marked adenoidal hyperplasia (white arrow). (b) Sagittal view showing marked adenoidal hyperplasia.

palate. The anterior aspect of the oropharynx begins at the circumvallate papillae and includes the posterior one-third of the tongue. Its lateral parameters are the palatine tonsils. The oropharyngeal mucosa and the constrictor muscles extend from the soft palate to the superior aspect of the epiglottis. The posterior oropharyngeal wall is related to C2 and C3, the second and third cervical vertebrae.

The pharynx is surrounded by visceral fascia surrounding its mucosa and muscu-lature, which acts as a barrier to contain tumor. If the fascia is violated, tumor may invade posteriorly into the longus capitis and colli muscles and the lower parapha-ryngeal space.

Simply stated, the skeletal support for the airway superiorly is the cranial base and associated pterygoid processes, posteriorly the cervical spine, anterosuperiorly the nasal cavity, and anteriorly the mandible and hyoid bone. Structures encroaching upon the airway include the nasal conchae, adenoids, soft palate, tongue, and the pharyngeal and lingual tonsils. Polyps and tumors may also contribute to obstruc-tion in an otherwise "open" system.

The Hypopharynx (Also Called Laryngopharynx)

The hypopharynx extends from the level of the hyoid bone to the cricopharyngeus, the lower level of the cricoids cartilage. According to Som and Curtin (2003), most authors divide the hypopharynx into the following three regions: the pyriform sinuses, the posterior wall, and the postcricoid region.

The pear-shaped pyriform sinus is situated on either side of the pharynx above by the inner surface of the thyrohyoid membrane and below by the thyroid cartilage and the lateral surface of the aryepiglottic fold. These two are referred to as the membranous and cartilaginous portions of the lateral pyriform sinus wall. The medial and posterior walls of the pyriform sinus are formed by the lateral surface of the aryepiglottic fold and the inferior continuation of the posterior wall of the oro-pharynx, respectively. The hypopharynx superior boundary is considered to be at the level of the hyoid bone. The posterior and lateral walls of the hypopharynx merge with the cricopharyngeus, which in turn merges with the cervical esophagus.

The postcricoid region is the anterior wall of the lower hypopharynx and is the interface between the hypopharynx and larynx. It extends from the level of the cri-coarytenoid joints down to the inferior aspect of the cricoids cartilage.

The Parapharyngeal Space

The parapharyngeal space is a dominant fat plane on either side of the pharynx that is best defined on T1-weighted images. Infiltration of the parapharyngeal space fat indicates deep invasion of a neoplasm.

On either side of the oropharyngeal airway are bilaterally symmetric soft-tissue masses, the tonsils and faucial pillars. Asymmetry in the size or configuration of these tonsils is an indication of possible tumor or infection presence on the enlarged side. A cystic enlargement of the palatine tonsil may indicate lymphoma, a tumor, or an abscess. Infection is generally associated with pain and malaise while a tumor causes little pain. It is not unusual to visualize dystrophic calcifications within the tonsillar crypts, and benign minor salivary gland retention cysts may occur.

References

The Sinonasal Cavity

Bent, J. P., Cuilty-Siller, C., Kuhn, F. A. (1994). The frontal cell as a cause of frontal sinus obstruction. *Am J Rhinology*, **8**, 185–91.

Gotwald, T. F., Zinreich, S. J., Corl, F., Fishman, E. K. (2001). Three-dimensional volumetric display of the nasal ostiomeatal channels and paranasal sinuses. *Am J Rhinology*, **176**, 241–45.

Huang, B. Y., Lloyd, K. M., DelGaudio J. M., et al. (2009). Failed endoscopic sinus surgery: spectrum of CT findings in the frontal recess. *Radiographics*, **29**(1), 177–95.

Som, P. M., and Curtin, H. D. (2003). *Head and Neck Imaging,* Volumes 1 and 2. Mosby.

The Pharynx

Harnsberger, H. (2006). *Diagnostic and Surgical Imaging Anatomy: Brain, Head and Neck, Spine (Diagnostic and Surgical Imaging Anatomy)*. Lippincott Williams & Wilkins.

Ikushima, I., Korogi, Y., Makita, O., Komohara, Y., Kawano, H., Yamura, M., Arikawa, K., Takahashi, M. (1999). MR imaging of Tornwaldt's cysts. *Am J Roentgenology*, **172**, 1663–5.

Netter, F. H. (2006). *Netter Atlas of Human Anatomy*, 4th ed. Saunders.

Ruprecht, A., and Dolan, K. D. (1991). The nasopharynx in oral and maxillofacial radiology. *Oral Surg, Oral Med, Oral Pathol*, **72**, 484–91.

Scarpace, S. L., et al. (2009). Treatment of head and neck cancers: issues for clinical pharmacists. *Pharmacotherapy*, **29**, 578–92.

Singal, R., et al. (1996). CT and MR imaging of squamous cell carcinoma of the tongue and floor of the mouth. *RadioGraphics*, **16**, 787–810.

Stambuk, H. E., et al. (2007). Oral cavity and oropharynx tumors. *Radiologic Clinics of North Am*, **47**, 1–20.

6

Cranial Skull Base and Orbits

Shawneen M. Gonzalez

Introduction

This chapter covers basic anatomy and common findings associated with the cranial skull base and orbits. The topics covered include anatomic variants/developmental anomalies and incidental findings. Different portions of the cranial skull base are seen on cone beam computed tomography (CBCT) scans depending on the field of view (FOV) used. Some of the radiographic findings covered in this chapter may not be visible on all scans.

Anatomy

This section highlights anatomical landmarks of the cranial skull base and orbits visualized on larger FOV scans. The cranial skull base is made up of the frontal bones, ethmoid bone, sphenoid bone, temporal bones, and occipital bone. The following table (Table 6.1) lists anatomical landmarks of the cranial skull base and the corresponding figures (Figures 6.1–6.15).

Interpretation Basics of Cone Beam Computed Tomography, Second Edition.
Edited by Shawneen M. Gonzalez.
© 2021 John Wiley & Sons, Inc. Published 2021 by John Wiley & Sons, Inc.
Companion website: www.wiley.com/go/gonzalez/interpretation

Table 6.1.   Cranial skull base anatomical landmarks with corresponding figure numbers.

Bone	Anatomical landmark	Axial	Coronal	Sagittal
Frontal	Frontal sinus (FS)	6.1	6.6	6.15
Ethmoid	Crista galli (CG)	6.1	6.7	
	Cribriform plate (CFP)		6.7	6.15
	Ethmoid air cells (EAC)	6.2	6.7	6.15
	Lamina papyracea (LP)	6.2	6.7	
Sphenoid	Anterior clinoid process (ACP)	6.2	6.8	6.14
	Sella turcica (ST)	6.2		6.15
	Posterior clinoid process (PCP)	6.2	6.9	6.15
	Sphenoid sinus (SS)		6.8	
	Pterygoid process (PP)	6.5	6.8	6.14
	Pterygopalatine fossa (PPF)	6.3 6.4		6.14
	Medial pterygoid plate (MPP)	6.4		
	Lateral pterygoid plate (LPP)	6.5		
	Clivus/basisphenoid (CB)	6.3		6.15
	Vidian canal (VC)	6.3	6.8	
	Foramen rotundum (FR)		6.8	
	Foramen lacerum (FL)*	6.3	6.9	
Temporal	Osseous external auditory canal (OEAC)	6.4	6.10	6.13
	Internal auditory canal (IAC)	6.3		
	Mastoid air cells (MAC)	6.3 6.4 6.5	6.10 6.11	6.12 6.13
	Petrous ridge (PR)	6.3	6.10 6.11	6.13
	Carotid canal (CC)	6.3		
	Styloid process (SP)	6.5		6.13
	Glenoid fossa (GF)	6.3	6.9	6.13
Occipital	Foramen magnum (FM)	6.4 6.5	6.11	6.15
	Jugular foramen (JF)		6.11	
	Occipital condyle (OC)			6.14
	Clivus/basiocciput (CO)	6.4 6.5	6.10	6.15

*The foramen lacerum is listed under the sphenoid bone but is at the junction of the sphenoid, temporal, and occipital bones.

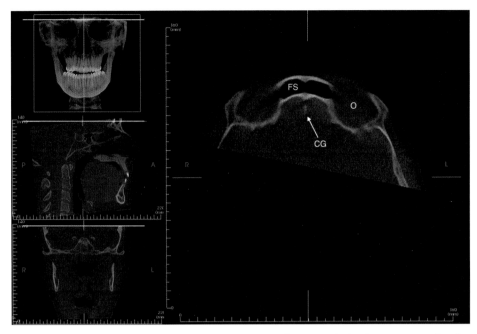

Figure 6.1. Axial view showing the frontal sinus (FS), crista galli (CG), and orbital cavities (O). Yellow line showing axial plane on left views (3D reconstruction, sagittal, and coronal).

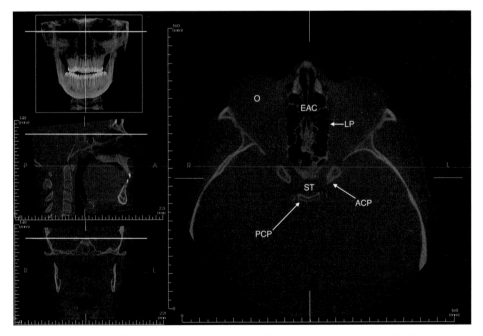

Figure 6.2. Axial view showing the ethmoid air cells (EAC), anterior clinoid process (ACP), sella turcica (ST), posterior clinoid process (PCP), lamina papyracea (LP), and orbital cavities (O). Yellow line showing axial plane on left views (3D reconstruction, sagittal, and coronal).

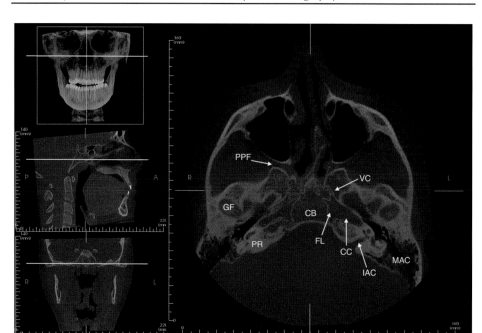

Figure 6.3. Axial view showing the pterygopalatine fossa (PPF), glenoid fossa (GF), petrous ridge (PR), clivus/basisphenoid (CB), foramen lacerum (FL), vidian canal (VC), carotid canal (CC), internal auditory canal (IAC), and mastoid air cells (MAC). Yellow line showing axial plane on left views (3D reconstruction, sagittal, and coronal).

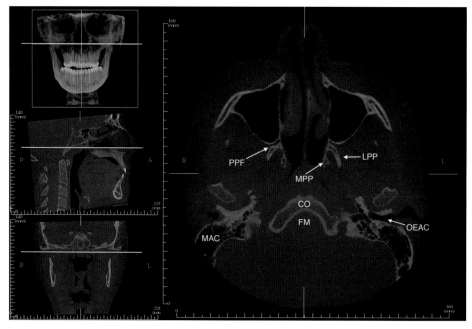

Figure 6.4. Axial view showing the pterygopalatine fossa (PPF), medial pterygoid plate (MPP), lateral pterygoid plate (LPP), clivus/occipital bone (CO), foramen magnum (FM), mastoid air cells (MAC), and osseous external auditory canal (OEAC). Yellow line showing axial plane on left views (3D reconstruction, sagittal, and coronal).

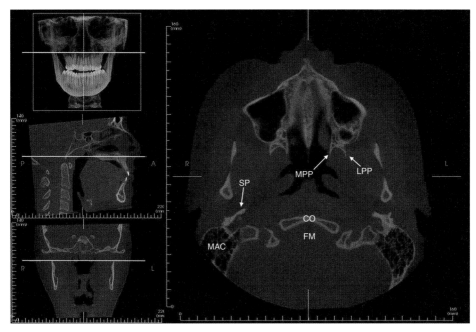

Figure 6.5.   Axial view showing lateral pterygoid plate (LPP), medial pterygoid plate (MPP), styloid process (SP), mastoid air cells (MAC), clivus/ basiocciput (CO), and foramen magnum (FM). Yellow line showing axial plane on left views (3D reconstruction, sagittal, and coronal).

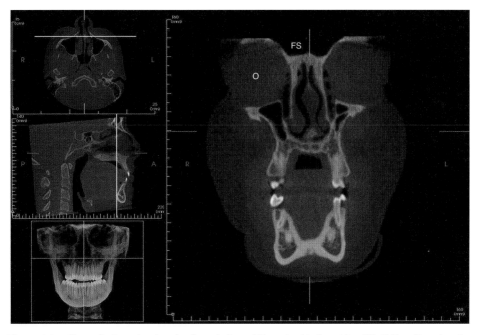

Figure 6.6.   Coronal view showing the frontal sinus (FS) and orbital cavities (O). Yellow line showing coronal plane on left views (axial and sagittal).

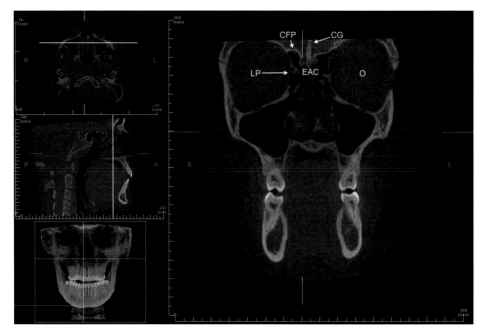

Figure 6.7.   Coronal view showing the cribriform plate (CFP), crista galli (CG), ethmoid air cells (EAC), lamina papyracea (LP), and orbital cavities (O). Yellow line showing coronal plane on left views (axial and sagittal).

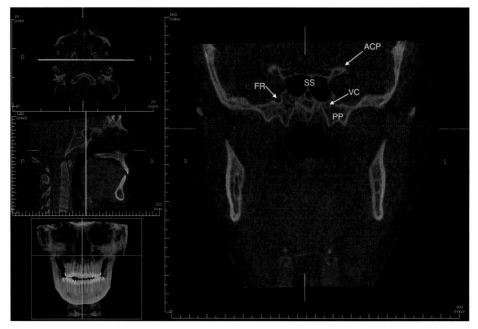

Figure 6.8.   Coronal view showing the foramen rotundum (FR), sphenoid sinus (SS), pterygoid process (PP), vidian canal (VC), and anterior clinoid process (ACP). Yellow line showing coronal plane on left views (axial and sagittal).

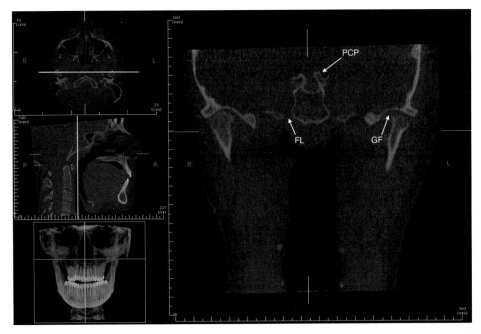

Figure 6.9. Coronal view showing the posterior clinoid process (PCP), foramen lacerum (FL), and glenoid fossa (GF). Yellow line showing coronal plane on left views (axial and sagittal).

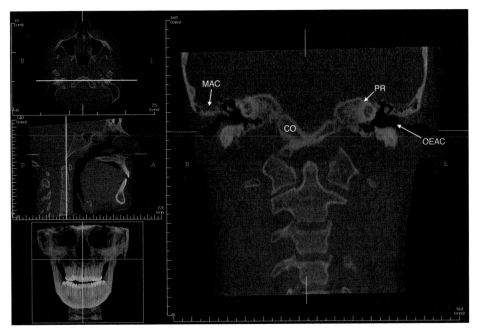

Figure 6.10. Coronal view showing the mastoid air cells (MAC), clivus/basiocciput (CO), petrous ridge (PR), and osseous external auditory canal (OEAC). Yellow line showing coronal plane on left views (axial and sagittal).

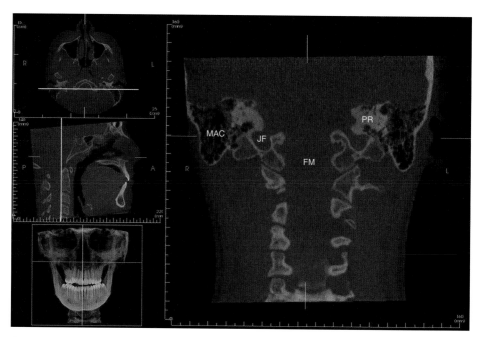

Figure 6.11. Coronal view showing the mastoid process with mastoid air cells (MAC), jugular foramen (JF), foramen magnum (FM), and petrous ridge (PR). Yellow line showing coronal plane on left views (axial and sagittal).

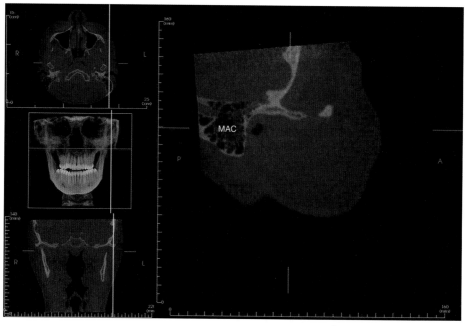

Figure 6.12. Sagittal view showing the mastoid process with mastoid air cells (MAC). Yellow line showing sagittal plane on left views (axial, 3D reconstruction, and coronal).

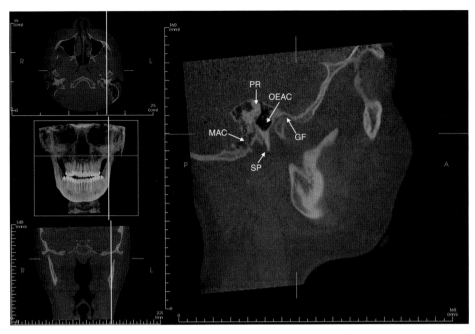

Figure 6.13. Sagittal view showing the mastoid air cells (MAC), petrous ridge (PR), osseous external auditory canal (OEAC), glenoid fossa (GF), and styloid process (SP). Yellow line showing sagittal plane on left views (axial, 3D reconstruction, and coronal).

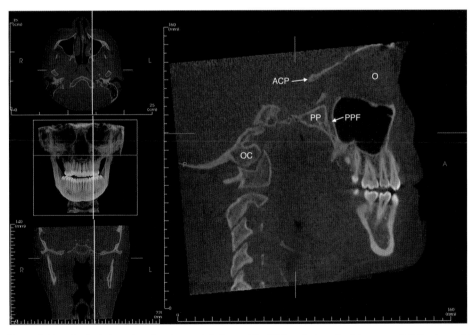

Figure 6.14. Sagittal view showing the occipital condyle (OC), anterior clinoid process (ACP), pterygoid process (PP), pterygopalatine fossa (PPF), and orbital cavity (O). Yellow line showing sagittal plane on left views (axial, 3D reconstruction, and coronal).

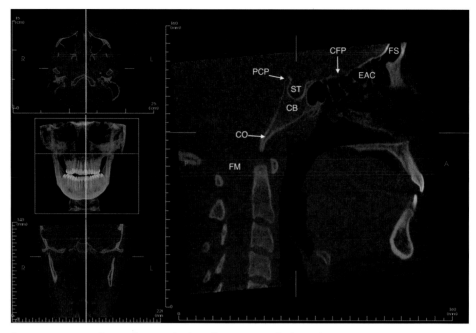

Figure 6.15. Sagittal view showing the frontal sinus (FS), cribriform plate (CFP), ethmoid air cells (EAC), sella turcica (ST), posterior clinoid process (PCP), clivus/basisphenoid (CB), clivus/basiocciput (CO), and foramen magnum (FM). Yellow line showing sagittal plane on left views (axial, 3D reconstruction, and coronal).

Anatomic Variants/Developmental Anomalies

Spheno-Occipital Synchondrosis (Basisphenoid-Basiocciput Synchondrosis)

Definition/Clinical Characteristics

The spheno-occipital synchondrosis is a developmental suture between the basiocciput of the occipital bone and basisphenoid of the sphenoid bone. The suture typically fuses near puberty (approximately between the ages of 11–16 for females and 12–18 for males) but may remain open until the age of 20.

Radiographic Description

This presents as a well-defined discontinuity separating the sphenoid and occipital bones. There may be no fusion to partial fusion of the suture (Figure 6.16) based on the age of the patient when scanned. This is best visualized on sagittal views (Figure 6.17) but is also visible on coronal and axial views (Figure 6.18).

Differential Interpretation

There is no differential interpretation due to the location, appearance, and age of patients.

Treatment/Recommendations

No further imaging or treatment is recommended if patient is under the age of 20.

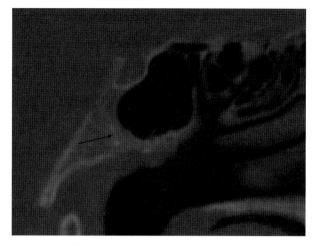

Figure 6.16.   Sagittal view on the midline showing the spheno-occipital synchondrosis with partial ossification (black arrow).

(a)   (b)

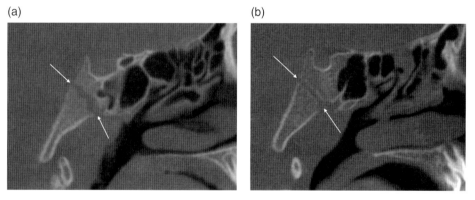

Figure 6.17.   (a) Sagittal view on the midline showing the spheno-occipital synchondrosis (white arrows). (b) Sagittal view on the midline showing the spheno-occipital synchondrosis (white arrows).

Cranial Thickness

Definition/Clinical Characteristics

The cranial thickness has a wide range of acceptable thicknesses. The cranial thickness does not correlate with the sex, age, or weight of an individual.

Radiographic Description

This presents as an equal thickness of the entire cranium (all bones visualized). The thickness can range from approximately 2 mm to 11 mm (Figures 6.19 and 6.20). The cranium will have intact cortical borders throughout all bones visualized. This is best visualized on axial views but is also visible on coronal and sagittal views.

(a)

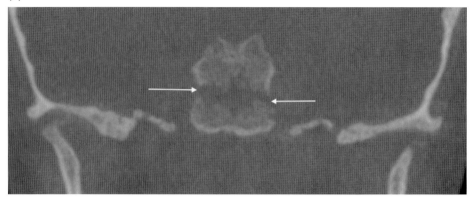

(b)

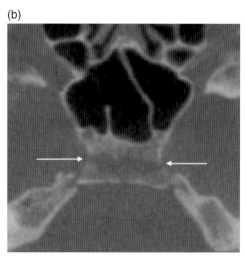

Figure 6.18.   (a) Coronal view at the mandibular condyles showing the spheno-occipital synchondrosis (white arrows). (b) Axial view showing the spheno-occipital synchondrosis (white arrows).

Differential Interpretation

If there is an uneven thickness (anterior posterior) of the frontal bone, the possibility of hyperostosis frontalis interna should be considered. Hyperostosis frontalis interna results in increased thickness of the frontal bone without affecting the other bones of the cranium. This is typically visualized superior to the orbits on axial views.

Treatment/Recommendations

No further imaging or treatment is recommended.

Vascular Markings

Definition/Clinical Characteristics

Vascular markings are indentations visible on the internal surface of the cranium created by blood vessels. There is no correlation with the presence of vascular markings and sex, age, or weight of an individual.

(a)

(b)

(c)

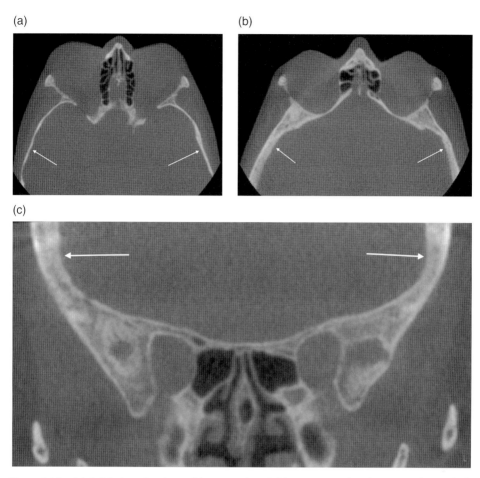

Figure 6.19.   (a) Axial view showing a thinner cranium (white arrows) within the range of normal. (b) Axial view showing a thicker cranium (white arrows) within the range of normal. (c) Coronal view showing a thicker cranium (white arrows) within the range of normal.

Radiographic Description

These present on any internal surface of the cranial skull base bones. They appear as well-defined, corticated radiolucent indentations of the cranial skull base. There is no universal shape for the markings (Figures 6.21 and 6.22). They may be unilateral or bilateral. These are visualized equally on all views (axial, coronal, and sagittal).

Differential Interpretation

There is no differential interpretation due to the location and appearance of this finding.

Treatment/Recommendations

No further imaging or treatment is recommended.

(a)

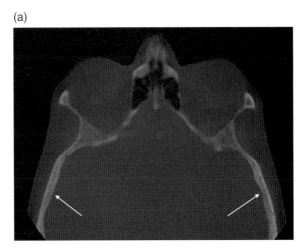

(b)

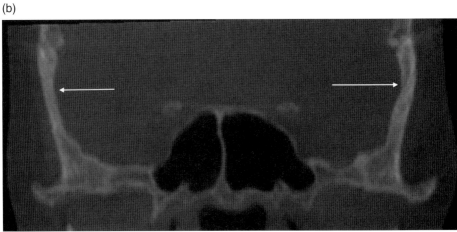

Figure 6.20. (a) Axial view showing cranial thickness within the range of normal (white arrows). (b) Coronal view showing a cranial thickness within the range of normal (white arrows).

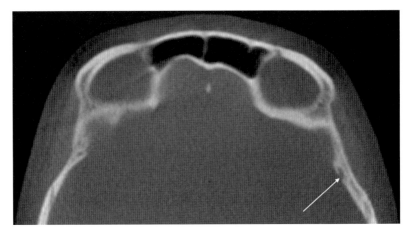

Figure 6.21. Axial view showing a radiolucent indentation on the internal surface of the cranium caused by vascular markings (white arrow).

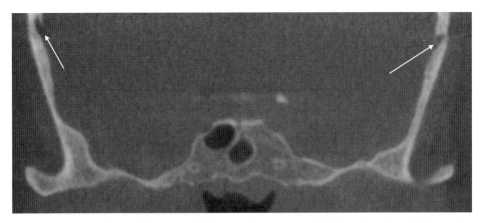

Figure 6.22. Coronal view showing radiolucent indentations on the internal surface of the cranium caused by vascular markings (white arrows).

Incidental Findings

Displacement of the Lamina Papyracea

Definition/Clinical Characteristics

The lamina papyracea is a thin bone on the medial border of the orbital cavity. It may protrude either medially from the orbit toward the ethmoid air cells or laterally into the orbit. Causes include trauma, iatrogenic and congenital reasons.

Radiographic Description

This presents as a displacement of the lamina papyracea medially or laterally. There may or may not be a discontinuity of the bone. Due to the nature of CBCT, it is not possible to determine if there is fat or muscle entrapment in this area. This is best visualized on axial and coronal views (Figures 6.23–6.25).

Differential Interpretation

There is no differential interpretation based on the location and appearance of this finding.

Treatment/Recommendations

Referral to primary care physician may be recommended for further investigation as this area is prone to increased risk during surgery.

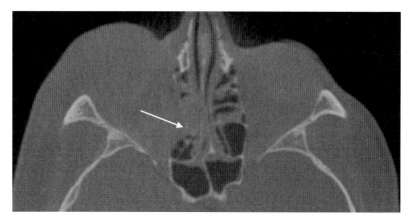

Figure 6.23.   Axial view showing medial displacement of the right lamina papyracea (white arrow).

(a)

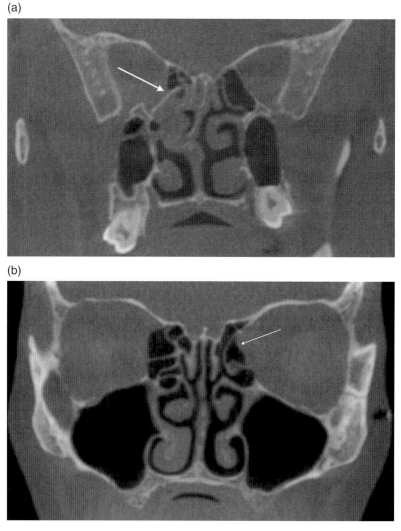

(b)

Figure 6.24.   (a) Coronal view showing medial displacement of the right lamina papyracea (white arrow). (b) Coronal view showing medial displacement of the left lamina papyracea (white arrow).

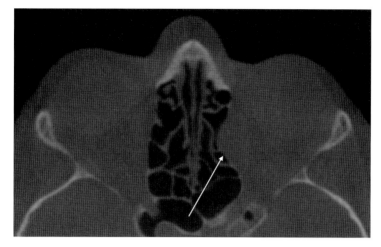

Figure 6.25.   Axial view showing medial displacement of the left lamina papyracea (white arrow).

References

Anatomy

Kennedy, T.A. Temporal bone. Learning Head and Neck. (https://www.learningheadandneck.com/anatomy/temporal-bone).

Netter, F. H. (2004). *Atlas of Human Anatomy*, 3d ed. Icon Learning Systems.

Anatomic Variants/Developmental Anomalies—Cranial Skull Base

Keats, T., and Anderson, M. (2007). *Atlas of Normal Roentgen Variants That May Simulate Disease*, 8th ed. Mosby.

Lynnerup, N. (2001). Cranial thickness in relation to age, sex and general body build in a Danish forensic sample. *Forensic Science International*, **117**, 45–51.

Ross, A. H., Jantz, R. L., McCormick, W. F. (1998). Cranial thickness in American females and males. *J Forensic Sciences*, **43**, 267–72.

Shirley, N. R., and Jantz, R. L. (2011). Spheno-occipital synchondrosis fusion in modern Americans. *J Forensic Sciences*, **56**, 580–5.

Incidental Findings—Orbits

Kendi, T. K., Rodrigez, C., Kemal, G., et al. (2004). Medial orbital wall protusion: computed tomography findings. *European J Radiology Extra*, **51**, 69–71.

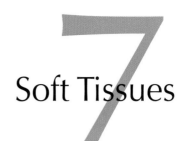

Soft Tissues

Shawneen M. Gonzalez

Introduction

This chapter covers no anatomy of the soft tissues because cone beam computed tomography (CBCT) is a hard-tissue imaging modality. All of the soft-tissue findings in this chapter are calcifications within the soft tissues. The topics covered include pathosis and incidental/other findings. Different portions of the soft tissue are seen on CBCT scans depending on the field of view (FOV) used. Some of the radiographic findings covered in this chapter may not be visible on all scans.

Pathosis—Arterial Calcifications

General Arterial Calcification Clinical Characteristics and Radiographic Findings

Arterial calcifications are strongly associated with existing systemic disease such as hypertension, hypercholesterolemia, and diabetes mellitus. There is a slight male predilection. Incidence increases with age. These are asymptomatic incidental findings.

Arterial calcifications have two different radiographic appearances. One type of calcification is arteriosclerosis (Monckeberg's medial calcinosis), which is calcifications of the lining of an artery. This presents radiographically with the outline of the artery visible. This more commonly occurs with intracranial arterial calcifications. The other type of calcification is calcified atherosclerotic plaque(s). These are plaques/masses that calcify on the internal walls of arteries. These first occur at arterial bifurcations such as the bifurcation of the internal and external carotid artery. These present radiographically as calcified masses, which may or may not be in a tube shape.

Interpretation Basics of Cone Beam Computed Tomography, Second Edition.
Edited by Shawneen M. Gonzalez.
© 2021 John Wiley & Sons, Inc. Published 2021 by John Wiley & Sons, Inc.
Companion website: www.wiley.com/go/gonzalez/interpretation

Internal (Cavernous) Carotid Artery Calcification

Definition/Clinical Characteristics

Calcifications of the internal carotid artery near the cavernous sinus. They are evident in approximately 10.6 % of the population on CBCT scans. There is suggestive correlation with intracranial arterial calcifications and strokes.

Radiographic Description

Calcification(s) present lateral to the sella turcica. They appear as well-defined radiopaque entities. The shape may present as either linear or a curved line on axial views (Figure 7.1) and sagittal views (Figure 7.2) to circular on coronal views (Figure 7.3). They may be unilateral or bilateral. Small plaques are more evident on coronal views, but calcifications may be seen on all views (Figure 7.4).

(a)   (b)

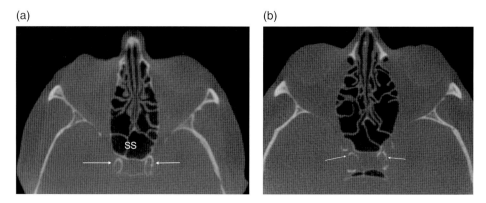

Figure 7.1.   (a) Axial view showing bilateral ovoid radiopaque lines (white arrows) consistent with cavernous carotid artery calcifications posterolateral to the sphenoid sinuses (SS). (b) Axial view showing bilateral linear radiopaque entities (white arrows) consistent with cavernous carotid artery calcifications.

(a)   (b)

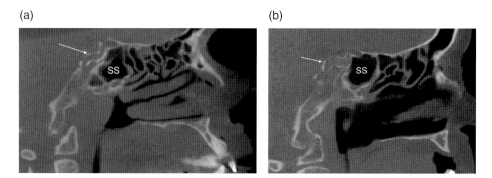

Figure 7.2.   (a) Sagittal view showing parallel curved radiopaque lines (white arrow) consistent with cavernous carotid artery calcification posterior to the sphenoid sinuses (SS). (b) Sagittal view showing parallel curved radiopaque lines (white arrow) consistent with cavernous carotid artery calcification posterior to the sphenoid sinuses (SS).

(a)

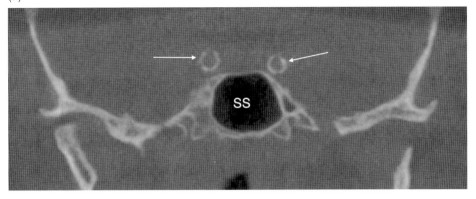

(b)

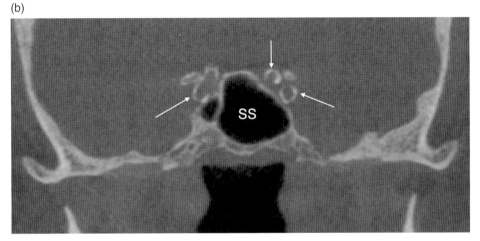

Figure 7.3. (a) Coronal view showing bilateral circular radiopaque entities (white arrows) consistent with cavernous carotid artery calcifications superolateral to the sphenoid sinus (SS). (b) Coronal view showing bilateral curved linear radiopaque entities (white arrows) consistent with cavernous carotid artery calcifications lateral to the sphenoid sinus (SS).

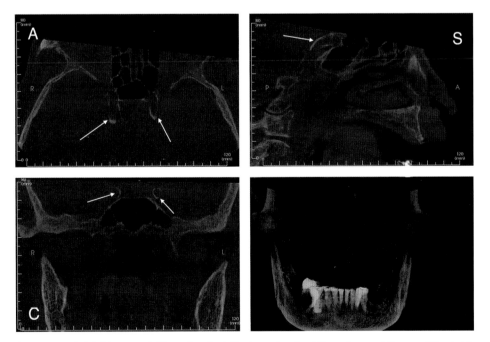

Figure 7.4. Axial (A), coronal (C), and sagittal (S) views showing bilateral curved linear entities (white arrows) consistent with cavernous carotid artery calcifications.

Differential Interpretation

There is no differential interpretation due to the location and appearance of this finding.

Treatment/Recommendations

Patients should be referred to their primary care physician. This ensures that the patient and primary care physician are aware of the full extent of any underlying atherosclerotic disease and/or other systemic disease contributing to the calcifications.

Vertebral Artery Calcification

Definition/Clinical Characteristics

Calcifications of the vertebral artery near the cranial skull base at the foramen magnum. They account for approximately 20% of intracranial arterial calcifications.

Radiographic Description

Calcification(s) present medial and posterior to the clivus and C1. They appear as well-defined radiopaque entities. The shape may present as either linear or a curved line on coronal views (Figure 7.5) and sagittal views (Figure 7.6) to circular on axial views (Figure 7.7). They may be unilateral or bilateral. Small plaques are more evident on axial views, but calcifications may be seen on all views (Figure 7.8).

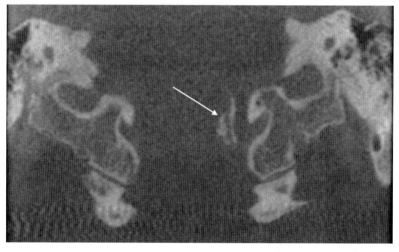

Figure 7.5. Coronal view showing parallel linear radiopaque entities (white arrow) in the foramen magnum consistent with left vertebral artery calcification.

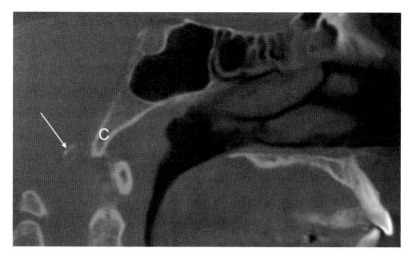

Figure 7.6. Sagittal view showing curved linear radiopaque entity (white arrow) in the foramen magnum consistent with vertebral artery calcification posterior to the clivus (C).

(a)

(b)

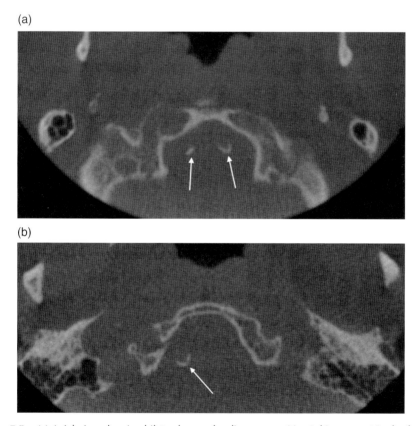

Figure 7.7. (a) Axial view showing bilateral curved radiopaque entities (white arrows) in the foramen magnum consistent with vertebral artery calcifications. (b) Axial view showing curved radiopaque entity (white arrow) in the foramen magnum consistent with right vertebral artery calcification.

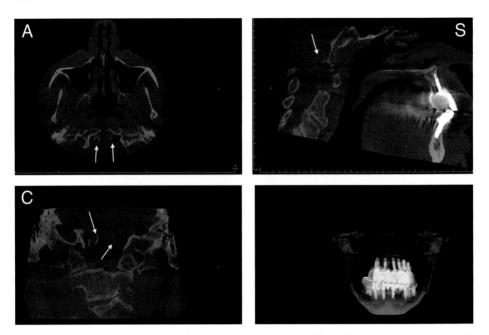

Figure 7.8.   Axial (A), coronal (C), and sagittal (S) views showing bilateral curved linear entities (white arrows) in the foramen magnum consistent with vertebral artery calcifications.

Differential Interpretation

There is no differential interpretation due to the location and appearance of this finding.

Treatment/Recommendations

Patient should be referred to their primary care physician. This ensures that the patient and primary care physician are aware of the full extent of any underlying atherosclerotic disease and/or other systemic disease contributing to the calcifications.

External Carotid Artery Calcification

Definition/Clinical Characteristics

Atherosclerotic plaques of the external carotid artery near the bifurcation of the internal and external carotid arteries. They are evident in approximately 5.5% to 10.4% of the population on CBCT scans covering this area.

Radiographic Description

Calcification(s) present antero-lateral to the junction of C3 and C4. They appear as well-defined radiopaque entities. They range in shape from linear and/or masses on coronal views (Figure 7.9) and sagittal views (Figure 7.10) to circular and/or masses on axial views (Figure 7.11). They may be unilateral or bilateral. Small plaques are more evident on axial views, but calcifications may be seen on all views (Figure 7.12).

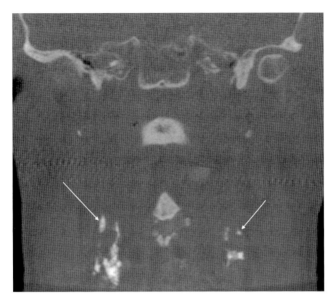

Figure 7.9. Coronal view showing multiple, bilateral radiopaque masses in a tube shape (white arrows) consistent with external carotid artery calcifications.

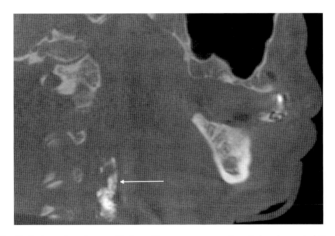

Figure 7.10. Sagittal view showing multiple radiopaque masses in a tube shape (white arrow) near the level of C3/C4 consistent with external carotid artery calcifications.

(a)   (b)

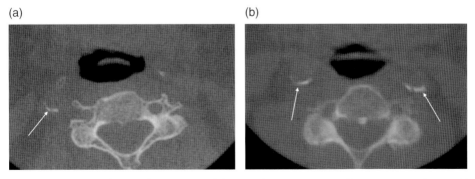

Figure 7.11. (a) Axial view showing curved linear radiopaque entity (white arrow) consistent with external carotid artery calcification. (b) Axial view showing bilateral curved linear radiopaque entities (white arrows) consistent with external carotid artery calcifications.

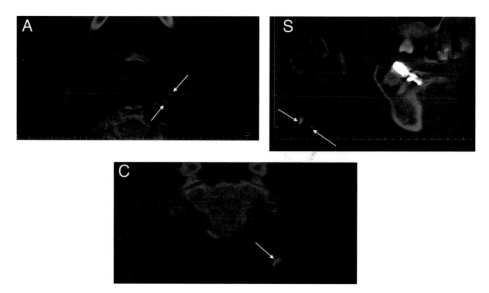

Figure 7.12. Axial (A), coronal (C), and sagittal (S) views showing left curved radiopaque entities (white arrows) consistent with external carotid artery calcifications.

Differential Interpretation

There is no differential interpretation due to the location and appearance of this finding.

Treatment/Recommendations

Patient should be referred to their primary care physician. This ensures that the patient and primary care physician are aware of the full extent of any underlying atherosclerotic disease and/or other systemic disease contributing to the calcifications.

Pathosis—Other Calcifications

Tonsiliths (Tonsilloliths, Tonsillar Calculi, Tonsillar Stones)

Definition/Clinical Characteristics

Tonsiliths are dystrophic calcifications of the tonsillar lymphoid tissues, most commonly associated with the palatine tonsils. These occur due to buildup of debris in the tonsillar crypts that calcify over time with repeated inflammation. They are frequently an incidental finding; however, there has been an association with halitosis noted. They have been noted in 1.3% to 24.6% of the population with an age range of 8 to 84 and a mean size of 2 mm to 4 mm.

Radiographic Description

They commonly present lateral to the airway. They appear as well-defined radiopaque entities ranging in shape from punctate entities to smooth/irregular masses (Figures 7.13 and 7.14). They may be unilateral or bilateral (Figure 7.15). They are visualized equally on all three views (axial, coronal, and sagittal).

(a)   (b)

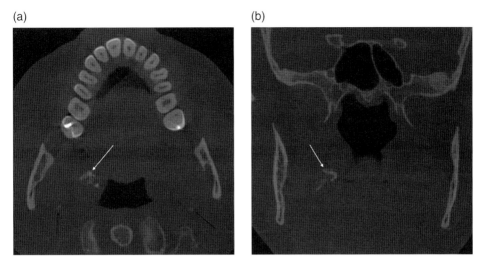

Figure 7.13.   (a) Axial view showing multiple well-defined radiopaque entities (white arrow) lateral to the airway consistent with tonsiliths and bilateral ossified stylohyoid ligaments (black arrows). (b) Coronal view showing multiple well-defined radiopaque entities (white arrow) consistent with tonsiliths.

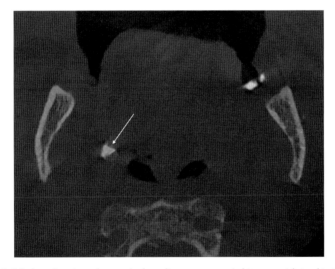

Figure 7.14.   Axial view showing a larger single radiopaque mass (white arrow) lateral to the airway consistent with a tonsilith.

Differential Interpretation

When the calcifications are further from the airway, an ossified stylohyoid ligament is a differential. An ossified stylohyoid ligament is circular and angled from the styloid process to the hyoid bone (Figure 7.13a).

Treatment/Recommendations

No further imaging or treatment is recommended for small tonsiliths. Larger tonsiliths may require referral for removal if the airway is compromised.

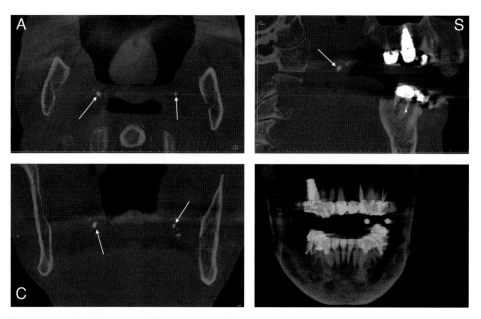

Figure 7.15. Axial (A), coronal (C), and sagittal (S) views showing multiple bilateral radiopaque entities (white arrows) lateral to the airway consistent with tonsiliths.

Sialolith

Definition/Clinical Characteristics

A dystrophic calcification within the salivary gland duct. It is more commonly noted in the Wharton's duct of the submandibular salivary gland. They are frequently associated with decreased salivary gland flow. Patients may present with pain and swelling in the floor of the mouth during mealtimes. They are found in 0.3% to 1.0% of CBCT scans.

Radiographic Description

A calcification that presents medial to the mandible in the floor of the mouth (submandibular salivary gland). They appear as a smooth to irregular, well-defined radiopaque mass (Figure 7.16). They may have a laminated appearance (Figure 7.17). They are typically unilateral. They are visualized equally on all three views (axial, coronal, and sagittal).

Differential Interpretation

There is no differential interpretation due to location.

Treatment/Recommendations

Recommend referral for further investigation of potential salivary flow issues and removal.

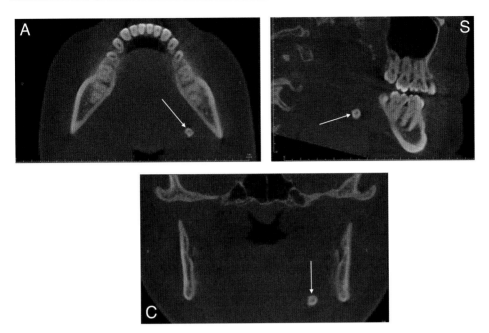

Figure 7.16. Axial (A), coronal (C), and sagittal (S) views showing a well-defined, round, radiopaque mass (white arrows) medial to the left posterior mandible in the floor of the mouth consistent with a sialolith.

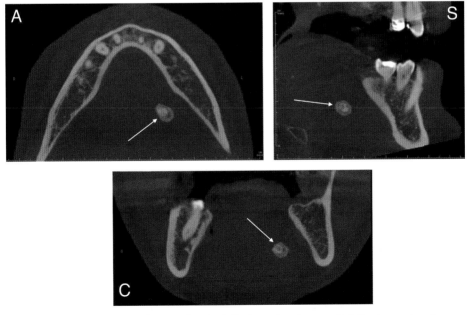

Figure 7.17. Axial (A), coronal (C), and sagittal (S) views showing a well-defined, round, radiopaque mass with laminations (white arrows) medial to the left posterior mandible in the floor of the mouth consistent with a sialolith.

Incidental Findings—Soft Tissue of the Brain

Pineal Gland Calcification

Definition/Clinical Characteristics

A physiological calcification of the pineal gland. Pineal gland calcification is the most common intracranial calcification. Pineal gland calcifications have been noted in 58.8% to 71.6% of the population. There is a male predilection. Populations exposed to increased sunlight and living at higher altitudes have shown decreased incidence of pineal gland calcification. Pineal gland calcification is frequently associated with choroid plexus calcification (Figure 7.18).

Radiographic Description

Calcification(s) appears in the midline superior to the foramen magnum. It appears as a well-defined radiopaque entity. The shape ranges from a punctate entity to multiple diffuse entities that combine to approximately 1 cm in diameter. Calcification is visualized equally on all three views (axial, coronal, and sagittal; Figures 7.19 and 7.20).

(a)   (b)

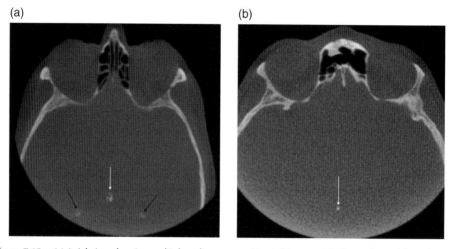

Figure 7.18.   (a) Axial view showing multiple radiopaque entities (white arrow) in the midline of the soft tissue of the brain consistent with pineal gland calcification and choroid plexus calcification as diffuse radiopaque areas (black arrows) lateral to the pineal gland calcification. (b) Axial view showing a single radiopaque entity (white arrow) in the midline of the soft tissue of the brain consistent with pineal gland calcification.

(a)   (b)

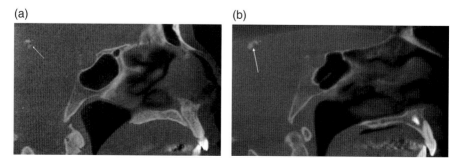

Figure 7.19.   (a) Sagittal view in the midline showing multiple radiopaque entities (white arrow) superior to the foramen magnum consistent with pineal gland calcification. (b) Sagittal view in the midline showing multiple radiopaque entities (white arrow) superior to the foramen magnum consistent with pineal gland calcification.

(a)   (b)

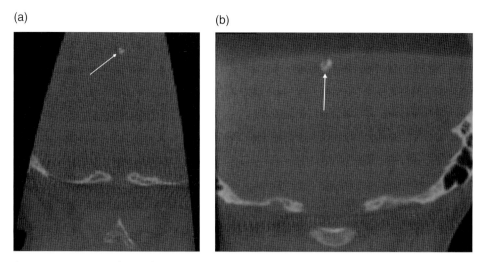

Figure 7.20.   (a) Coronal view showing multiple radiopaque entities (white arrow) in the midline of the soft tissue of the brain consistent with pineal gland calcification. (b) Coronal view showing multiple radiopaque entities (white arrow) in the midline of the soft tissue of the brain consistent with pineal gland calcification.

Differential Interpretation

Based on the location and size, there is no other differential interpretation of patients over the age of 7. When multiple calcifications are noted in patients under the age of 7 or are larger than 1 cm in diameter, a neoplastic process of the pineal gland cannot be ruled out.

Treatment/Recommendations

If found in a patient under the age of 7 or larger than 1 cm in diameter, referral to a primary care physician is recommended for further investigation of a possible neoplastic origin.

No further imaging or treatment is recommended on patients over the age of 7.

Choroid Plexus Calcification

Definition/Clinical Characteristics

Physiological calcifications of the choroid plexus most commonly present in the atria of the lateral ventricles. These are incidental findings. The incidence increases with age, occurring in approximately 2.6% to 70.2% of the population.

Radiographic Description

Calcification(s) present in the posterior aspect of the soft tissue of the brain. They appear as diffuse radiopaque entities lateral to the midline (Figure 7.21). They are either unilateral or bilateral. They are more commonly visualized on axial and coronal views (Figure 7.22) but may be seen on all views (Figure 7.23).

Differential Interpretation

There are no differential interpretations based on the location and appearance of this finding.

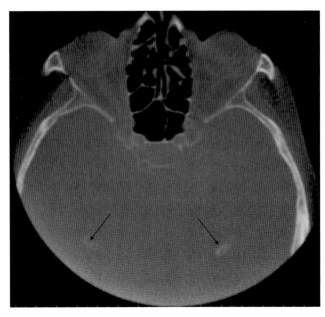

Figure 7.21.   Axial view showing bilateral diffuse radiopaque areas (black arrows) consistent with choroid plexus calcifications.

(a)   (b)

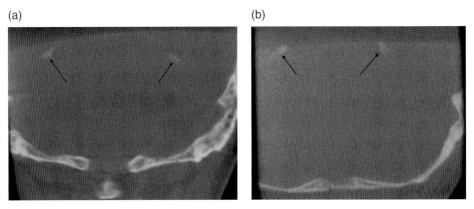

Figure 7.22.   (a) Coronal view showing bilateral diffuse radiopaque areas (black arrows) consistent with choroid plexus calcifications. (b) Coronal view showing bilateral diffuse radiopaque areas (black arrows) consistent with choroid plexus calcifications.

Treatment/Recommendations

No further imaging or treatment is recommended.

Dural Calcifications

Definition/Clinical Characteristics

Physiologic calcifications of the dura of the brain. These are incidental findings occurring in approximately 10% to 12.5% of the population. There is a male predilection.

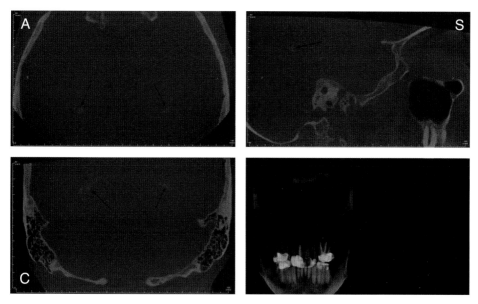

Figure 7.23.   Axial (A), coronal (C), and sagittal (S) views showing bilateral diffuse radiopaque areas (black arrows) consistent with choroid plexus calcifications.

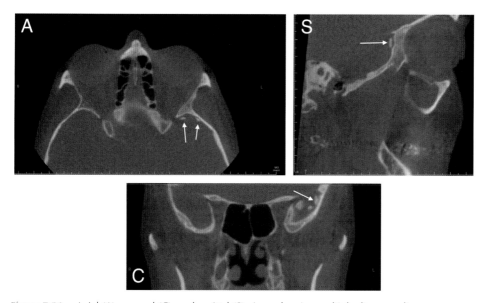

Figure 7.24.   Axial (A), coronal (C), and sagittal (S) views showing multiple, linear, radiopaque masses adjacent to the cranial skull base (white arrows) consistent with dural calcifications.

Radiographic Description

Calcification(s) present adjacent to the cranium or in the midline. They range in shape from linear radiopaque entities (Figure 7.24) to radiopaque masses (Figure 7.25). They may be found in the midline or adjacent to the cranium. They are visualized equally on all three views (axial, coronal, and sagittal; Figure 7.26).

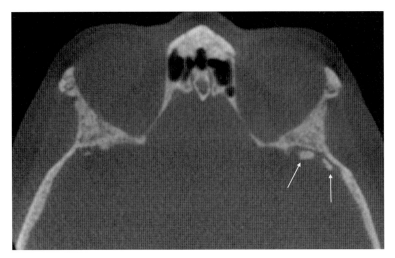

Figure 7.25.   Axial view showing multiple radiopaque masses adjacent to the cranial skull base (white arrows) consistent with dural calcifications.

(a)

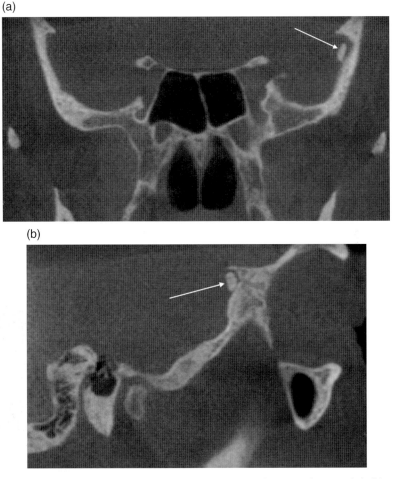

(b)

Figure 7.26.   (a) Coronal view showing a single radiopaque mass adjacent to the cranial skull base (white arrow) consistent with a dural calcification. (b) Sagittal view showing a single radiopaque mass adjacent to the cranial skull base (white arrow) consistent with a dural calcification.

Differential Interpretation

There are no differential interpretations based on the location and appearance of this finding.

Treatment/Recommendations

No further imaging or treatment is recommended.

Interclinoid Ligament Calcification

Definition/Clinical Characteristics

A calcification of the ligament attached to the anterior and posterior clinoid processes of the sella turcica. There is no clinical significance of this finding; however, it has been noted as an incidental finding in basal cell nevus syndrome. The incidence of complete calcification of the ligament ranges from 4% to 19% of the population; however, these studies were performed on lateral cephalometric skull radiographs and not computed tomography (CT) images.

Radiographic Description

It appears as a well-defined, radiopaque line between the anterior and posterior clinoid processes of the sella turcica. There may be partial calcification to complete calcification (Figure 7.27) connecting the two processes (anterior to posterior). It may be either unilateral or bilateral. This is most evident on sagittal and axial views (Figure 7.28).

Differential Interpretation

There is no differential interpretation due to the location and appearance of this finding.

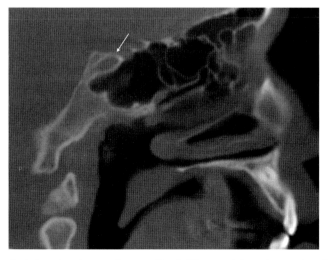

Figure 7.27. Sagittal view showing a radiopaque line (white arrow) from the anterior clinoid process to the posterior clinoid process consistent with complete calcification of the interclinoid ligament.

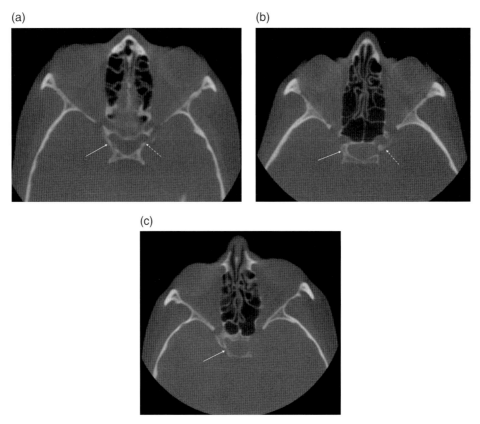

Figure 7.28.   (a) Axial view showing bilateral interclinoid ligament calcification. There is complete calcification on the right (white arrow) and near complete calcification on the left (white dashed arrow). (b) Axial view showing bilateral interclinoid ligament calcification. There is complete calcification on the right (white arrow) and near complete calcification on the left (white dashed arrow). (c) Axial view showing right complete interclinoid ligament calcification (white arrow).

Treatment/Recommendations

No further imaging or treatment is recommended.

Petroclinoid Ligament Calcification

Definition/Clinical Characteristics

A physiological calcification of the ligament extending from the posterior clinoid process to the petrous ridge of the temporal bone. This an incidental finding noted in approximately 2.6% of the population. There is no clinical significance of this finding; however, it has been noted as an incidental finding in basal cell nevus syndrome.

Radiographic Description

It appears as a well-defined, radiopaque line between the posterior clinoid process of the sella turcica and the petrous ridge of the temporal bone. There may be partial to complete calcification (Figures 7.29 and 7.30). It may be either unilateral or bilateral. This is most evident on sagittal and axial views.

(a) (b)

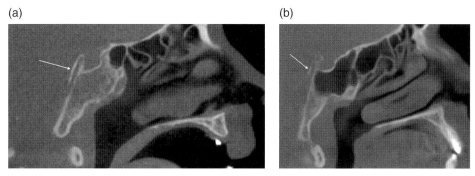

Figure 7.29. (a) Sagittal view showing a radiopaque line (white arrow) extending inferiorly from the posterior clinoid process consistent with partial petroclinoid ligament calcification. (b) Sagittal view showing a radiopaque line (white arrow) extending inferiorly from the posterior clinoid process consistent with partial petroclinoid ligament calcification.

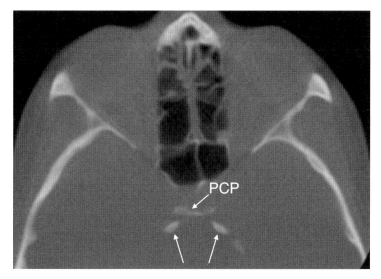

Figure 7.30. Axial view showing bilateral petroclinoid ligament calcification (white arrows) posterior to the posterior clinoid process (PCP).

Differential Interpretation

There is no differential interpretation due to the location and appearance of this finding.

Treatment/Recommendations

No further imaging or treatment is recommended.

Incidental Findings—Orbital Cavity

Scleral Plaques

Definition/Clinical Characteristics

Physiological calcifications of the sclera. This is an incidental finding noted in approximately 3% of CT scans of patients 60 years and older. Incidence increases with age.

Radiographic Description

Calcification(s) located at the insertion sites of the medial and lateral rectus muscles to the globe. They present as linear radiopaque entities (Figure 7.31) to small masses. They may be unilateral or bilateral per globe. They may affect one or both globes. They are visualized on all views (axial, coronal, and sagittal; Figures 7.32 and 7.33).

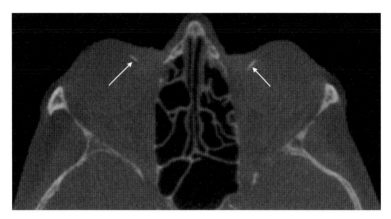

Figure 7.31.   Axial view showing bilateral curved linear radiopaque entities at the medial aspect of the globes (white arrows) consistent with scleral plaques.

(a)

(b)

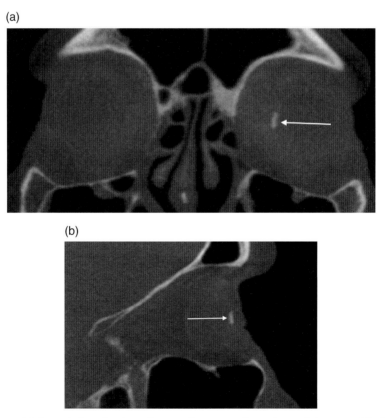

Figure 7.32.   (a) Coronal view showing a linear radiopaque entity at the medial aspect of the left globe (white arrow) consistent with a scleral plaque. (b) Sagittal view showing a linear radiopaque entity on the globe (white arrow) consistent with a scleral plaque.

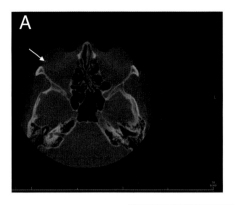
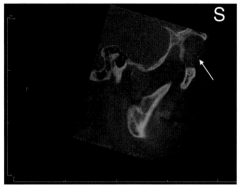
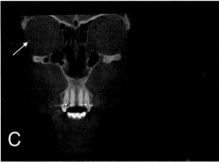

Figure 7.33.   Axial (A), coronal (C), and sagittal (S) views showing a punctate radiopaque entity on the lateral aspect of the right globe (white arrows) consistent with a scleral plaque.

Differential Interpretation

Calcifications noted on the globe not at the insertion point of the muscles may indicate macular degeneration, infection, inflammation, or trauma.

Treatment/Recommendations

No further imaging or treatment is recommended.

Trochlear Apparatus Calcification

Definition/Clinical Characteristics

The trochlear apparatus is a cartilaginous loop that allows the movement of the superior oblique muscle. It is located at the supero-medial aspect of the orbital rim. This is an incidental finding occurring in approximately 16% of the population. There is a male predilection.

Radiographic Description

Calcification(s) found at the superior-medial aspect of the orbital rim near the anterior aspect (Figure 7.34). They present as a well-defined, curved linear radiopaque entity (Figure 7.35). It may be unilateral or bilateral. They are visualized equally on all three views (axial, coronal, and sagittal).

Differential Interpretation

There is no differential interpretation due to the location and appearance of this finding.

(a)

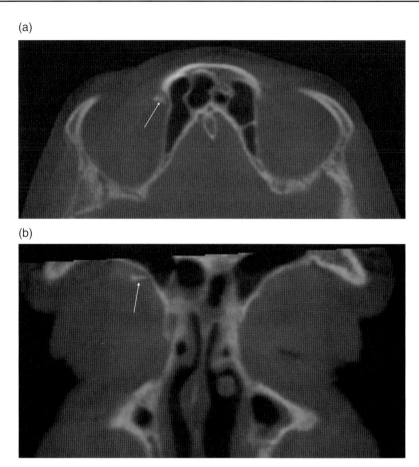

(b)

Figure 7.34. (a) Axial view showing a curved radiopaque entity in the right orbital cavity (white arrow) consistent with calcification of the trochlear apparatus. (b) Coronal view showing a linear radiopaque entity at the supero-medial aspect of the right orbital cavity (white arrow) consistent with trochlear apparatus calcification.

Treatment/Recommendations

No further imaging or treatment is recommended.

Incidental Findings—Face

Osteoma Cutis

Definition/Clinical Characteristics

Ossification in the superficial soft tissue of the skin. Some patients may have a history of acne. This is an incidental finding noted in approximately 1% to 2.3% of CBCT scans. These are not clinically visible on the skin.

Radiographic Description

Calcification(s) present in the skin. They appear as punctate, well-defined radiopaque entities (Figure 7.36). It may be unilateral or bilateral (Figure 7.37). They are visualized equally on all three views (axial, coronal, and sagittal).

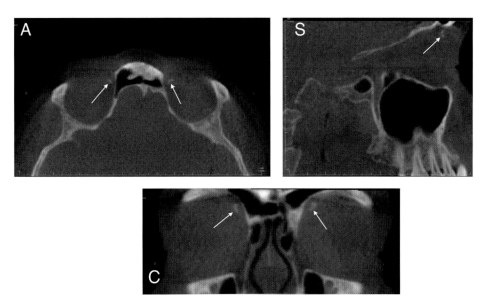

Figure 7.35.   Axial (A), coronal (C), and sagittal (S) views showing bilateral curved radiopaque entities at the supero-medial aspects of the right and left orbital cavity consistent with trochlear apparatus calcifications.

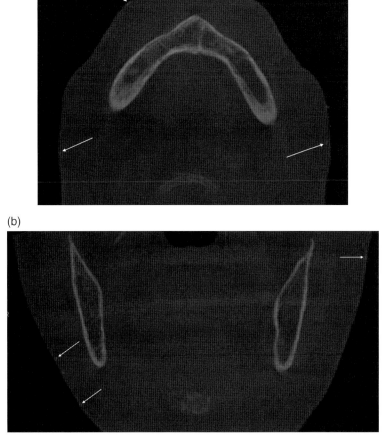

Figure 7.36.   (a) Axial view showing multiple punctate radiopaque entities (white arrows) in the superficial soft tissue of the skin consistent with osteoma cutis. (Not all areas identified with arrows.) (b) Coronal view showing multiple punctate radiopaque entities (white arrows) in the superficial soft tissue of the skin consistent with osteoma cutis. (Not all areas identified with arrows.)

(a)

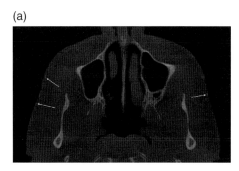

(b)

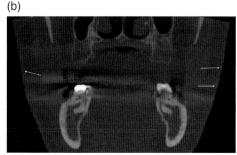

Figure 7.37.   (a) Axial view showing multiple radiopaque entities (white arrows) in the superficial soft tissue of the skin consistent with osteoma cutis. (Not all areas identified with arrows.) (b) Coronal view showing multiple radiopaque entities (white arrow) in the superficial soft tissue of the skin consistent with osteoma cutis. (Not all areas identified with arrows.)

Differential Interpretation

Cases with multiple sites of osteoma cutis (hundreds or more) are referred to as multiple miliary osteoma cutis.

There is no differential interpretation due to the location and appearance of this finding.

Treatment/Recommendations

No further imaging or treatment is recommended.

References

Pathosis — Arterial Calcifications

Babiarz, L. S., Yousem, D. M., Bilker, W., et al. (2005). Middle cerebral artery infarction: relationship of cavernous carotid artery calcification. *Am J Neuroradiol*, **26**, 1505–11.

Babiarz, L. S., Yousem, D. M., Wasserman, B. A., et al. (2003). Cavernous carotid artery calcification and white matter ischemia. *Am J Neuroradiol*, **24**, 872–7.

Barghan, S., Tahmasbi Arashlow, M., Nair, M. K. (2016). Incidental findings on cone beam computed tomography studies outside of the maxillofacial skeleton. *Int J Dent.* **2016**, 9196503.

Kiroglu, Y., Calli, C., Karabulut, N., et al. (2010a). Intracranial calcifications on CT. *Diagn Interv Radiol*, **16**, 263–9.

Pette, G. A., Norkin, F. J., Ganeles, J., et al. (2012). Incidental findings from a retrospective study of 318 cone beam computed tomography consultation reports. *Int J Oral Maxillofac Implants*, **27**, 595–603.

Ptak, T., Hunter, G. H., Avakian, R., et al. (2003). Clinical significance of cavernous carotid calcifications encountered on head computed tomography scans performed on patients seen in the emergency department. *J Computer Assisted Tomography*, **27**, 505–9.

Pathosis — Other Calcifications

Fauroux, M.-A., Mas, C., Tramini, P. et. al. (2013). Prevalanece of palatine tonsilloliths: a retrospective study on 150 consecutive CT examinations. *Dentomaxillofac Radiol*, **42**, 2012049.

Koenig, L. (Ed.). (2012). *Diagnostic Imaging: Oral and Maxillofacial Radiology*. Amirsys.

Mallaya, S., and Lam, E. (Ed.). (2019a) *White and Pharaoh's Oral Radiology: Principles and Interpretation*. Mosby.

Yalcin, E. D., Ararat, E. (2020). Prevalence of soft tissue calcifications in the head and neck region: a cone-beam computed tomography study. *Niger J Clin Pract*, **23**, 759–63.

Incidental Findings / Other—Soft Tissue of the Brain

Admassie, D., and Mekonnen, A. (2009). Incidence of normal pineal and choroid plexus calcification on brain CT (computed tomography) at TikurAnbessa Teaching Hospital Addis Ababa, Ethiopia. *Ethiop Med J*, **47** (1), 55–60.

Cederberg, R. A., Benson, B. W., Nunn, M., et al. (2003). Calcification of the interclinoid and petroclinoid ligaments of sella turcica: a radiographic study of the prevalence. *Orthodontic Craniofacial Research*, **6**, 227–32.

Doyle, A. J., and Anderson, G. D. (2006). Physiologic calcification of the pineal gland in children on computed tomography: prevalence, observer reliability and association with choroid plexus calcification. *Acad Radiol*, **13**, 822–26.

Kiroglu, Y., Calli, C., Karabulut, N., et al. (2010b). Intracranial calcifications on CT. *Diagn Interv Radiol*, **16**, 263–9.

Mutalik, S., and Tadinada, A. (2017). Prevalence of pineal gland calcification as an incidental finding in patients referred for implant dental therapy. *Imaging Sci Dent*, **47**, 175–80.

Sedghizadeh, P. P., Nguyen, M., Enciso, R. (2012). Intracranial physiological calcifications evaluated with cone beam CT. *Dentomaxillofac Radiol*, **41**, 675–8.

Turgut, A. T., Karakas, H. M., Ozsunar, Y., et al. (2008). Age-related changes in incidence of pineal gland calcification in Turkey: a prospective multicenter CT study. *Pathophysiology*, **15**, 41–48.

Incidental Findings/Other—Orbital Cavity

Ko, S. J., and Kim, Y. J. (2010). Incidence of calcification of the trochlear apparatus in the orbit. *Korean J Opthalmol*, **24** (1), 1–3.

LeBedis, C. A., and Sakai, O. (2008). Nontraumatic orbital conditions: diagnosis with CT and MR imaging in the emergent setting. *RadioGraphics*, **28**, 1741–53.

Murray, J. L., Haymany, L. A., Tang, R. A., et al. (1995). Incidental asymptomatic orbital calcifications. *J Neuroophthalmol*, **15**, 203–8.

Incidental Findings/Other—Face

Alhazmi, D., Badr, F., Jadu, F., et. al. (2017). Osteoma cutis of the face in CBCT images. *Case Rep Dent*, **2017**, 8468965.

Mallaya, S., and Lam, E. (Ed.). (2019b). *White and Pharaoh's Oral Radiology: Principles and Interpretation*. Mosby.

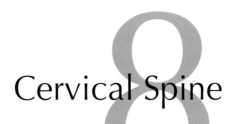

Cervical Spine

Shawneen M. Gonzalez

Introduction

This chapter covers basic anatomy and common findings associated with the cervical spine. The topics covered include anatomic variants/developmental anomalies and pathosis. Different portions of the cervical spine are seen on cone beam computed tomography (CBCT) scans depending on the field of view (FOV) used. Some of the radiographic findings covered in this chapter may not be visible on all scans.

Anatomy

This section highlights anatomical landmarks of the cervical vertebrae visualized on larger FOV scans. The first three to four cervical vertebrae are the most commonly visualized vertebrae on CBCT scans (Figures 8.1–8.10).

C1 (Atlas)

The superior most vertebra, C1, is a ring-shaped vertebra composed of an anterior and posterior arch with bilateral transverse processes between the two. There is no body of C1.

Interpretation Basics of Cone Beam Computed Tomography, Second Edition.
Edited by Shawneen M. Gonzalez.
© 2021 John Wiley & Sons, Inc. Published 2021 by John Wiley & Sons, Inc.
Companion website: www.wiley.com/go/gonzalez/interpretation

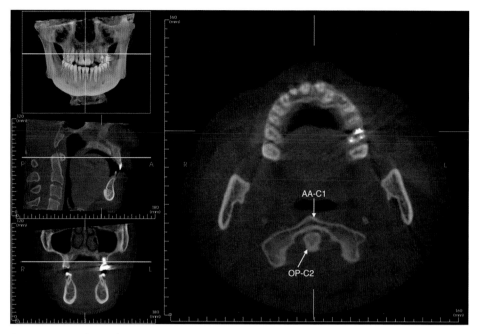

Figure 8.1.   Axial view showing the anterior arch of C1 (AA-C1) and the odontoid process of C2 (OP-C2). Yellow line showing axial plane on left views (3D reconstruction, sagittal, and coronal).

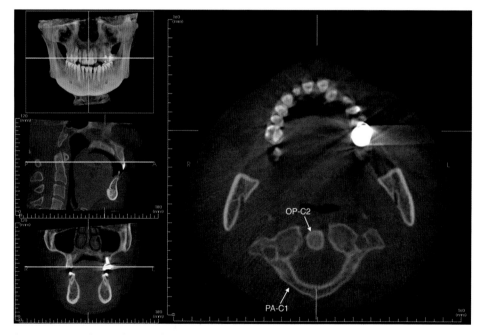

Figure 8.2.   Axial view showing the odontoid process of C2 (OP-C2) and posterior arch of C1 (PA-C1). Yellow line showing axial plane on left views (3D reconstruction, sagittal, and coronal).

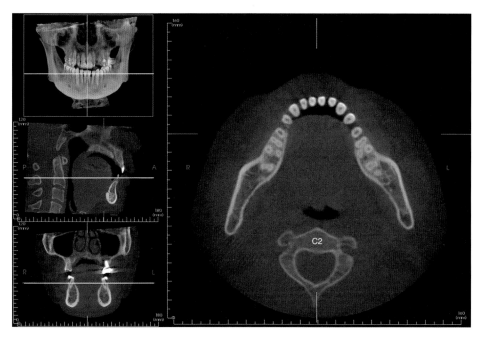

Figure 8.3. Axial view showing the entire arch of C2. Yellow line showing axial plane on left views (3D reconstruction, sagittal, and coronal).

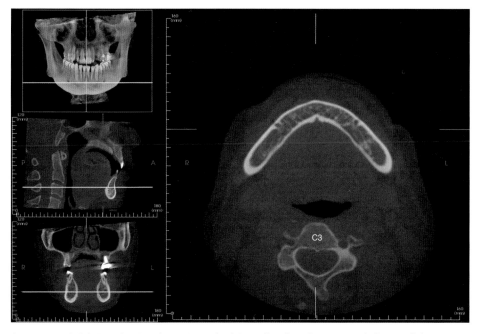

Figure 8.4. Axial view showing the entire arch of C3. Yellow line showing axial plane on left views (3D reconstruction, sagittal, and coronal).

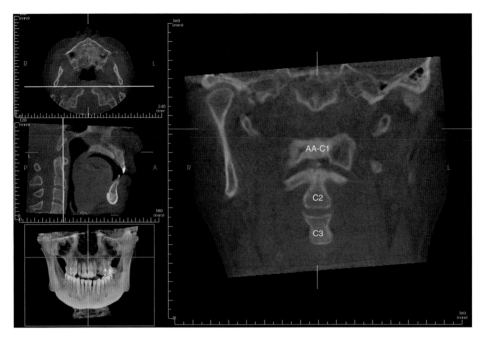

Figure 8.5. Coronal view showing the anterior arch of C1 (AA-C1) and portions of the body of C2 and C3. Yellow line showing coronal plane on left views (axial and sagittal).

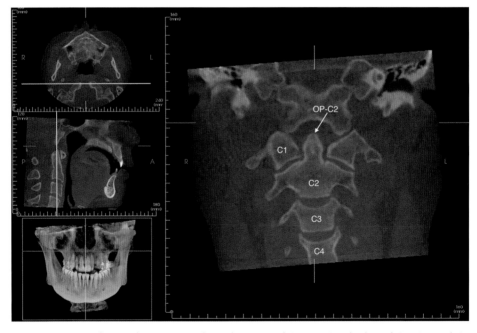

Figure 8.6. Coronal view showing C1, odontoid process of C2 (OP-C2), bodies of C2, C3, and C4. Yellow line showing coronal plane on left views (axial and sagittal).

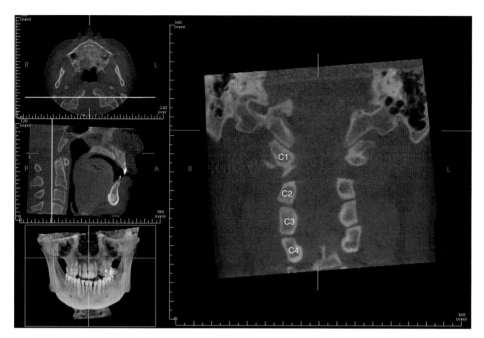

Figure 8.7. Coronal view showing transverse processes of C1, C2, C3, and C4. Yellow line showing coronal plane on left views (axial and sagittal).

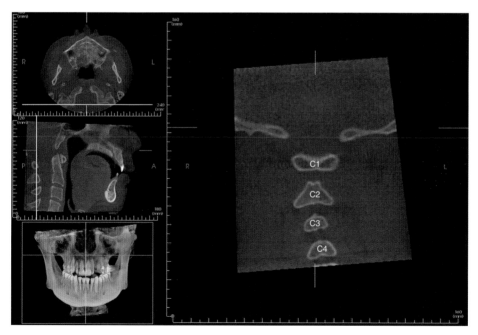

Figure 8.8. Coronal view showing the posterior arch of C1 and spinous processes of C2, C3, and C4. Yellow line showing coronal plane on left views (axial and sagittal).

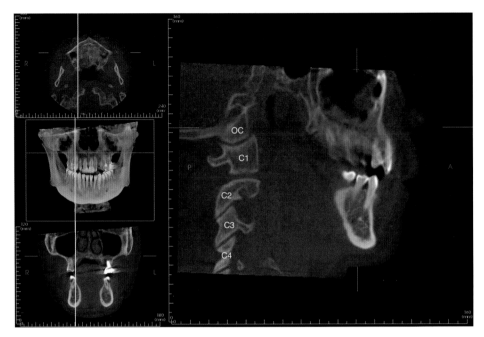

Figure 8.9. Sagittal view showing the occipital condyle (OC) and transverse process of C1, C2, C3, and C4. Yellow line showing sagittal plane on left views (axial, 3D reconstruction, and coronal).

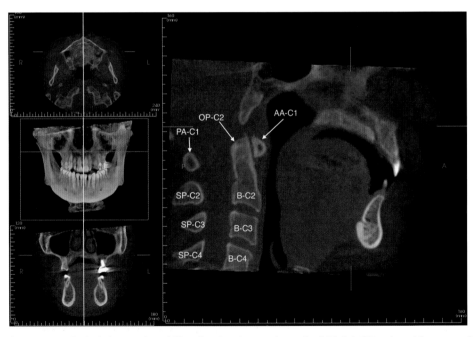

Figure 8.10. Sagittal view on the midline showing the anterior arch of C1 (AA-C1), odontoid process of C2 (OP-C2), posterior arch of C1 (PA-C1), bodies of cervical vertebrae C2 (B-C2), C3 (B-C3), C4 (B-4), and spinous processes of C2 (SP-C2), C3 (SP-C3), C4 (SP-C4). Yellow line showing sagittal plane on left views (axial, 3D reconstruction, and coronal).

C2 (Axis)

The second cervical vertebra is composed of a body (anteriorly) with the addition of a superior projection (odontoid process) that sits posterior to the anterior arch of C1. The remaining components of the vertebra are transverse processes and a spinous process (posteriorly) creating a ring where the spinal cord courses through.

C3–C7

The remaining vertebrae are composed of a body (anteriorly), transverse processes, and a spinous process (posteriorly) creating a ring where the spinal cord courses through.

Anatomic Variants/Developmental Anomalies

Clefts (C1)

Definition/Clinical Characteristics

Clefts are incomplete fusions of the ossification centers of the cervical spine. They present either at the anterior or posterior arch of C1 (atlas) or a combination of both (split atlas). The fusion of the anterior arch occurs by the age of 10 and the posterior arch between the ages of 3 and 4. Posterior arch clefts have an incidence of 4% of all adults, with 97% of these clefts occurring in the midline. Anterior arch clefts are less common, occurring in only 0.1% of all adults. Cervical vertebral clefts occur more commonly in patients with cleft lip, cleft palate, or both.

Radiographic Description

It presents as a well-defined, corticated discontinuity of the anterior or posterior arch of C1. There may be multiple discontinuities (three or more) in the anterior arch (Figure 8.11). The posterior arch rarely presents with more than one discontinuity. It is best visualized on axial and coronal views (Figures 8.12–8.14).

(a)   (b)

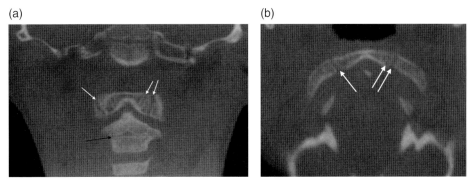

Figure 8.11. (a) Coronal view showing three anterior arch clefts (white arrows) of C1 and partial subdental synchrondrosis of C2 (black arrow). (b) Axial view showing three anterior arch clefts (white arrows) of C1.

(a)   (b)

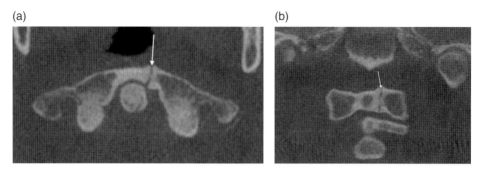

Figure 8.12.   (a) Axial view showing a single anterior arch cleft (white arrow) of C1. (b) Coronal view showing a single anterior arch cleft (white arrow) of C1.

(a)   (b)

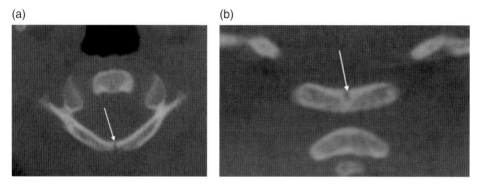

Figure 8.13.   (a) Axial view showing a single posterior arch cleft (white arrow) of C1. (b) Coronal view showing a single posterior arch cleft (white arrow) of C1.

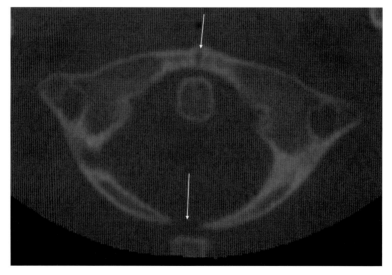

Figure 8.14.   Rotated axial view showing an anterior arch cleft and posterior arch cleft of C1 (white arrows) consistent with a split atlas.

Differential Interpretation

A discontinuity with no cortication should include a differential of a fracture. A fracture typically presents with swelling combined with a history of trauma to the area.

Treatment/Recommendations

No further imaging or treatment is recommended.

Os Terminale (C2)

Definition/Clinical Characteristics

There are three ossification centers that fuse to form the body of C2 (axis). Two create the body and one the tip of the odontoid process. The ossification center that forms the tip of the odontoid process is referred to as os terminale. It is typically evident by the age of 3 and fuses with the body of C2 by the age of 12.

Radiographic Description

This presents as a well-defined, corticated bony fragment at the tip of the body of C2. The body of C2 presents with a V-shaped notch on the superior aspect where the ossification center is located on coronal views (Figure 8.15). There may be a complete to incomplete separation of the ossification center from the remainder of the body of C2. It is best visualized on coronal and sagittal views (Figure 8.16).

Differential Interpretation

If the ossification center is evident beyond the age of 12, it is referred to as ossiculum terminale persistens. A fracture of the tip of the odontoid process will also present as a bony fragment separated from the body of C2. The bony fragment and body will not have corticated borders at the area of separation. A history of trauma indicates a fracture more likely than a persistent ossification center.

(a)   (b)

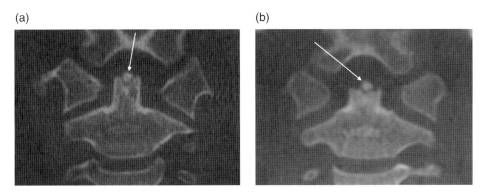

Figure 8.15.   (a) Coronal view showing os terminale (white arrow) at the superior aspect of the odontoid process of C2. (b) Coronal view showing os terminale (white arrow) at the superior aspect of the odontoid process of C2.

(a)   (b)

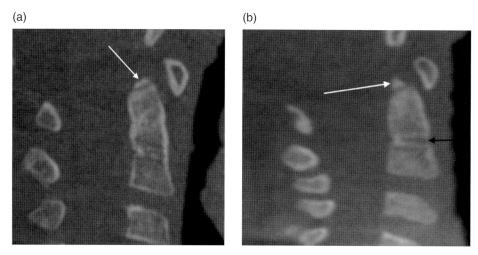

Figure 8.16. (a) Sagittal view showing os terminale (white arrow) at the superior aspect of the odontoid process of C2. (b) Sagittal view showing os terminale (white arrow) at the superior aspect of the odontoid process of C2 and subdental synchondrosis (black arrow) of C2.

Treatment/Recommendations

No further imaging or treatment is recommended.

Subdental Synchondrosis (C2)

Definition/Clinical Characteristics

Subdental synchondrosis is the developmental suture between two ossification centers that make the body of C2. Fusion occurs in 80% of the population by the age of 9. Persistence of the synchondrosis is referred to as a "dentocentral ghost."

Radiographic Description

This appears as a horizontal radiolucent line or band in the middle of the C2 body. It may extend completely from one side to the other (anterior–posterior or laterally; Figure 8.17a) or only partially (Figures 8.11a, 8.16b, 8.17b) depending on the stage of fusion. Complete separation of the two ossification centers is typically not seen beyond the age of 4. It is best visualized on sagittal and coronal views (Figure 8.18).

Differential Interpretation

A fracture of the C2 body in this location can occur; however, the presence of swelling along with a history of trauma to this area would rule out persistent synchondrosis.

Treatment/Recommendations

No further imaging or treatment is recommended.

(a)

(b)

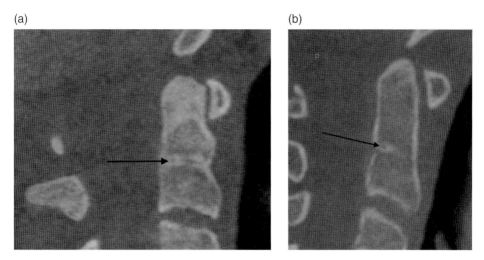

Figure 8.17.   (a) Sagittal view showing complete subdental synchondrosis (black arrow) of C2. (b) Sagittal view showing partial subdental synchondrosis (black arrow) of C2.

(a)

(b)

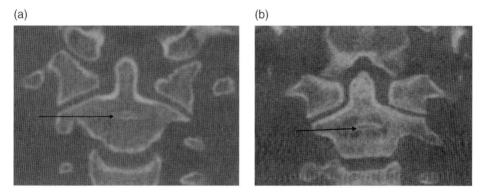

Figure 8.18.   (a) Coronal view showing partial subdental synchondrosis (black arrow) of C2. (b) Coronal view showing partial subdental synchondrosis (black arrow) of C2.

Congenital Block Vertebrae (Non-segmentation)

Definition/Clinical Characteristics

Congenital block vertebrae is the failure of separation of two or more adjacent vertebral bodies or transverse processes. This occurs in 5.5% of the population.

Radiographic Description

This most commonly occurs at the C2-C3 junction. It presents at the bodies, right, and/or left transverse processes. An enlarged body and/or transverse process with the absence of a radiolucent disc space is evident (Figure 8.19). It is best visualized on sagittal and coronal views (Figure 8.20).

Differential Interpretation

Fusion of C2 and C3 vertebra is associated with type 2 Klippel–Feil syndrome (KFS). These patients may present with scoliosis (60%) or have limited range of motion, specifically lateral bending of the spine (more commonly seen in patients with 4+

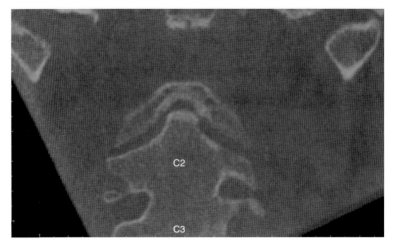

Figure 8.19.   Coronal view showing congenital block vertebrae of the bodies of C2 and C3.

(a)   (b)

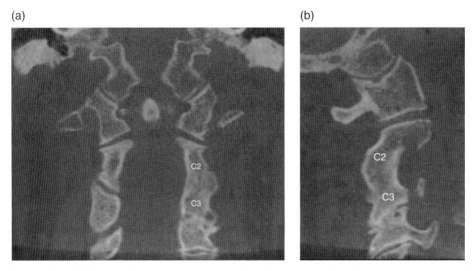

Figure 8.20.   (a) Coronal view showing congenital block vertebrae of the left transverse processes of C2 and C3. (b) Sagittal view showing congenital block vertebrae of the left transverse processes of C2 and C3.

vertebrae fused). Many patients are asymptomatic throughout their entire life. KFS occurs in approximately 1 in 40,000–42,000 births.

Fusion may occur in cases of severe degenerative joint disease changes. The vertebrae will show other signs of degenerative joint disease changes (Figure 8.23) in these situations.

Treatment/Recommendations

Referral to the patient's primary care physician may be recommended to evaluate for the presence of KFS.

Degenerative Joint Disease (Osteoarthritis, Spondylosis)

Definition/Clinical Characteristics

Degenerative joint disease (DJD) is a common age-related disease process resulting in degenerative changes of the intervertebral joints. DJD affects 50% of the population over the age of 40, increasing to 85% of the population over the age of 60. Activities or occupations that involve increased loads on the cervical vertebrae increase the risk of developing DJD. Patients with DJD of the cervical vertebrae may be asymptomatic or have a range of symptoms including neck pain, cervical radiculopathy, and cervical myelopathy. There is a wide range of classifications of DJD; however, we will only cover the radiographic classifications in this book.

Radiographic Description

There are five basic radiographic findings associated with DJD: asymmetrical intervertebral joint spacing narrowing, osteophyte formation, bone erosions, subchondral cysts, and facet hypertrophy.

Asymmetrical Intervertebral Joint Space Narrowing

The radiolucent intervertebral joint spaces should appear uniform in size (Figure 8.21). Asymmetrical joint space narrowing is one of the first signs of DJD (Figures 8.22 and 8.23). Evaluating the joint spaces is best visualized on sagittal views.

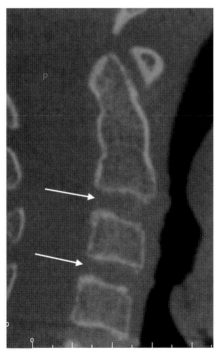

Figure 8.21. Sagittal view on midline showing normal intervertebral joint spacing between the bodies of C2-C3-C4 (white arrows).

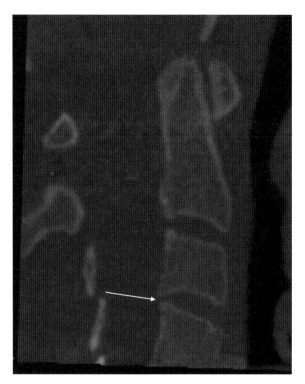

Figure 8.22.   Sagittal view on midline showing asymmetrical intervertebral joint space narrowing (white arrow) between the bodies of C3-C4.

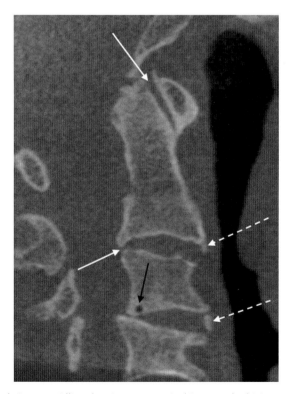

Figure 8.23.   Sagittal view on midline showing asymmetrical intervertebral joint space narrowing (white arrows), osteophyte formation (white dashed arrows), and subchondral cyst formation (black arrow).

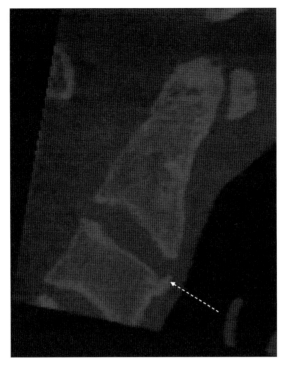

Figure 8.24.   Sagittal view on midline showing osteophyte formation (white dashed arrow) of C3.

Osteophyte Formation

Osteophytes form in an attempt to increase stability of the cervical vertebrae. They appear as bone spurs at the junctions of the vertebrae and intervertebral joint spaces (Figures 8.23 and 8.24). They grow and enlarge toward the adjacent vertebra. They may increase in size such that they impinge on the spinal cord, producing myeloradiculopathy. They are best visualized on sagittal views.

Bone Erosions

Bone erosions appear on the surfaces of the vertebra in direct contact with the intervertebral joint space. They appear as a discontinuity of the cortical border with saucering and loss of the bone in this area. They are best visualized on sagittal and coronal views (Figure 8.25).

Subchondral Cysts

Subchondral cysts are degenerative cysts that form at the junctions of the vertebrae and intervertebral joint spaces. They appear as well-defined, round/ovoid radiolucent areas within the vertebra (Figures 8.23 and 8.26). They are visualized on all three views equally (axial, coronal, and sagittal).

Facet Hypertrophy

Facet hypertrophy is an increase in bone formation at the facet between two adjacent vertebrae. It appears as bony enlargement of the junction of transverse processes. It is best visualized on axial views (Figures 8.27 and 8.28).

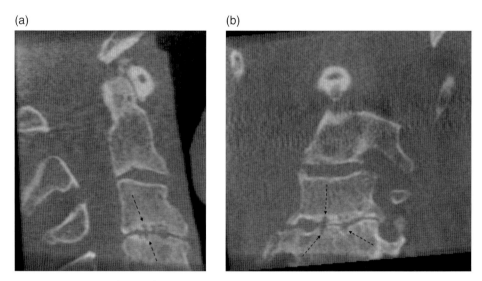

Figure 8.25.   (a) Sagittal view showing bone erosions between the bodies of C3 and C4 (black dashed arrows). (b) Coronal view showing bone erosions between the bodies of C3 and C4 (black dashed arrows).

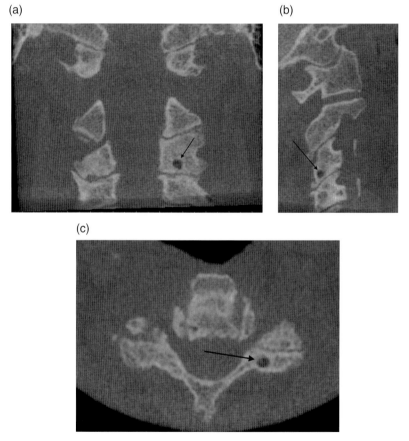

Figure 8.26.   (a) Coronal view showing subchondral cysts in the left transverse process of C3 (black arrow). (b) Sagittal view showing subchondral cysts in the left transverse process of C3 (black arrow). (c) Axial view showing subchondral cysts in the left transverse process of C3 (black arrow).

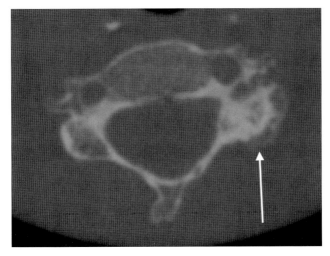

Figure 8.27. Axial view showing left facet hypertrophy (white arrow).

(a)   (b)

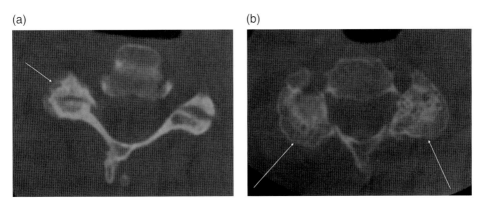

Figure 8.28. (a) Axial view showing right facet hypertrophy (white arrow). (b) Axial view showing bilateral facet hypertrophy (white arrows).

Luoma et al. (2009) classified spinal DJD in four groups ranging from Grade 0 to Grade 3. The classification is based on the presence or absence of the five previous radiographic findings (Table 8.1).

Differential Interpretation

There is no differential interpretation due to the presence of multiple pathognomic radiographic findings of this disease process.

Treatment/Recommendations

Patients should be referred to their primary care physician. The primary care physician will determine whether treatment is necessary.

Table 8.1 Radiographic degenerative joint disease (DJD) classification.

Radiographic finding	Grade 0 (no radiographic DJD)	Grade 1 (mild radiographic DJD)	Grade 2 (moderate radiographic DJD)	Grade 3 (severe radiographic DJD)
Asymmetrical joint space narrowing	None present	Present	Present	Present
Osteophytes	None present	Small	Small	Large
Bone erosions	None present	None present	Mild	Severe
Subchondral cysts	None present	None present	Small	Large
Facet hypertrophy	None present	None present	Moderate	Severe

Source: Based on Luoma et al. (2009).

References

Anatomy

Netter, F. H. (2004). *Atlas of Human Anatomy*, 3d ed. Icon Learning Systems.

Anatomic Variants/Developmental Anomalies

Bertozzi, J. C., Rojas, C. A., Martinez, C. R. (2009). Evaluation of the pediatric craniocervical junction on MDCT. *AJR*, **192**, 26–31.

De Graaff, R. (1982). Congenital block vertebrae C2-C3 in patients with cervical myelopathy. *Acta Neurochir*, **61** (1–3), 111–26.

Karwacki, G. M., and Schneider, J. F. (2012). Normal ossification patterns of atlas and axis: a CT study. *Am J Neuroradiol*, **33**, 1882–7.

Keats, T., and Anderson, M. (2007). *Atlas of Normal Roentgen Variants That May Simulate Disease*, 8th ed. Mosby.

Klimo, P., Rao, G., Brockmeyer, D. (2007). Congenital anomalies of the cervical spine. *Neurosurg Clin N Am*, **18**, 463–78.

Knoplich, J. (1992). Isolated vertebral blocks in the cervical spine. *Rev Paul Med*, **110** (1), 2–7.

Piatt, J. H., and Grissom, L. E. (2011). Developmental anatomy of the atlas and axis in childhood by computed tomography. *J Neurosurg Pediatrics*, **8**, 235–43.

Popat, H., Drage, N., Durning, P. (2008). Mid-line clefts of the cervical vertebrae— an incidental finding arising from cone beam computed tomography of the dental patient. *Br Dent J*, **204**, 303–6.

Samartzis, B., Lubicky, J. P., Shen, F. H. (2008). "Bone block" and congenital spine deformity. *Ann Acad Med Singapore*, **37**, 624.

Smoker, W. R. K. (1994). Craniovertebral junction: normal anatomy, craniometry, and congenital anomalies. *RadioGraphics*, **14**, 255–77.

Viswanathan, A., Whitehead, W. E., Luerssen, T. G., et al. (2009). "Orthotopic" ossiculum terminale persistens and atlantoaxial instability in a child less than 12 years of age: a case report and review of the literature. *Cases Journal*, **2**, 8530–5.

Pathosis

Leonardi, M., Simonetti, L., Agati, R. (2002). Neuroradiology of spine degenerative disease. *Best Practice & Research Clinical Rheumatology*, **16** (1), 59–87.

Luoma, K., Vehmas, T., Grönblad, M., et al. (2009). Relationship of Modic type 1 change with disc degeneration: a prospective MRI study. *Skeletal Radiol*, **38**, 237–44.

Narayan, P., and Haid, R. W. (2001). Treatment of degenerative cervical disc disease. *Neurologic Treatment*, **19** (1), 217–29.

Rao, R. D., Currier, B. L., Albert, T. J., et al. (2007). Degenerative cervical spondylosis: clinical syndromes, pathogenesis, and management. *J Bone Joint Surg Am*, **89**, 1360–78.

Maxilla and Mandible (excluding TMJs)

Shawneen M. Gonzalez

Introduction

This chapter covers basic anatomy and common findings associated with the maxilla and mandible. The topics covered include anatomic variants/developmental anomalies, pathosis, and incidental/other findings. Different portions of the maxilla and mandible are seen on cone beam computed tomography (CBCT) scans depending on the field of view (FOV) used. Some of the radiographic findings covered in this chapter may not be visible on all scans.

Anatomy

This section highlights anatomical landmarks of the maxilla and mandible, excluding the temporomandibular joints (TMJs - see chapter 10). Table 9.1 lists anatomical landmarks and the corresponding figures (Figures 9.1–9.10).

Interpretation Basics of Cone Beam Computed Tomography, Second Edition.
Edited by Shawneen M. Gonzalez.
© 2021 John Wiley & Sons, Inc. Published 2021 by John Wiley & Sons, Inc.
Companion website: www.wiley.com/go/gonzalez/interpretation

Table 9.1. Maxilla and mandible anatomical landmarks with corresponding figure numbers.

Bone	Anatomical landmark	Axial	Coronal	Sagittal
Maxilla	Nasopalatine canal (NPC)	9.1	9.5	9.10
	Incisive foramen (IF)	9.2	9.5	9.10
Mandible	Mandibular foramen (MNF)	9.2	9.8	
	Inferior alveolar nerve canal (IAN)	9.3	9.7	9.9
	Mental foramen (MF)	9.4	9.6	9.9
	Genial tubercle (GT)	9.4		9.10

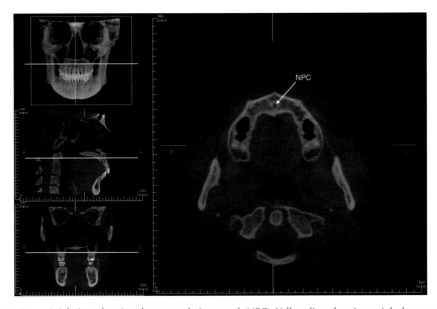

Figure 9.1. Axial view showing the nasopalatine canal (NPC). Yellow line showing axial plane on left views (3D reconstruction, sagittal, and coronal).

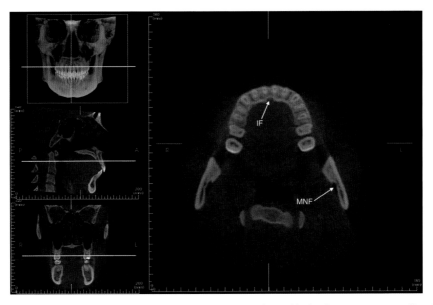

Figure 9.2. Axial view showing the incisive foramen (IF) and mandibular foramen (MNF). Yellow line showing axial plane on left views (3D reconstruction, sagittal, and coronal).

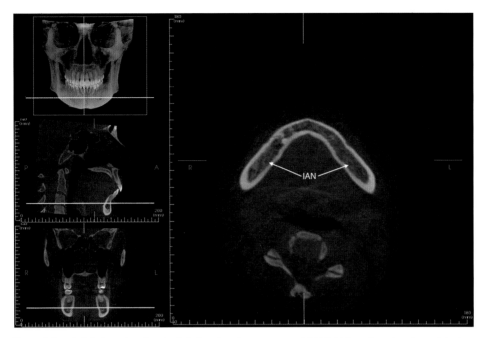

Figure 9.3. Axial view showing the inferior alveolar nerve canal (IAN). Yellow line showing axial plane on left views (3D reconstruction, sagittal, and coronal).

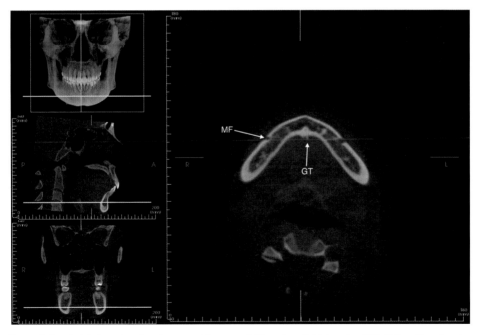

Figure 9.4. Axial view showing the mental foramen (MF) and genial tubercles (GT). Yellow line showing axial plane on left views (3D reconstruction, sagittal, and coronal).

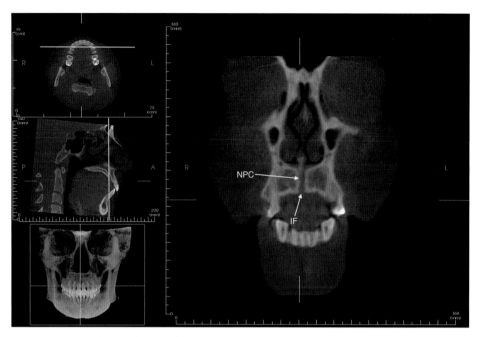

Figure 9.5.   Coronal view showing the nasopalatine canal (NPC) with the incisive foramen (IF) at the inferior aspect. Yellow line showing coronal plane on left views (axial and sagittal).

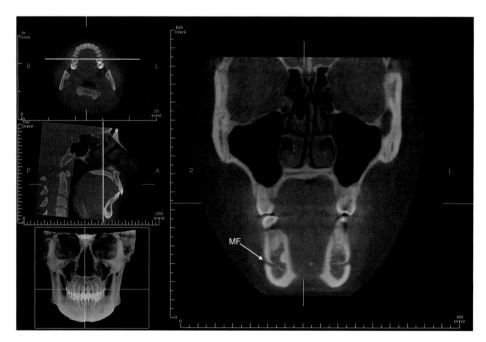

Figure 9.6.   Coronal view showing the mental foramen (MF). Yellow line showing coronal plane on left views (axial and sagittal).

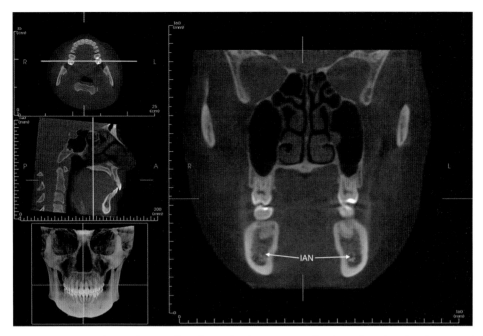

Figure 9.7. Coronal view showing the inferior alveolar nerve canal (IAN). Yellow line showing coronal plane on left views (axial and sagittal).

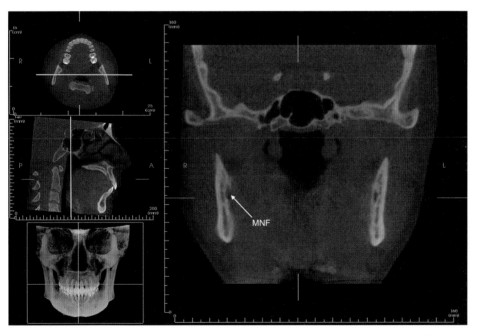

Figure 9.8. Coronal view showing the mandibular foramen (MNF). Yellow line showing coronal plane on left views (axial and sagittal).

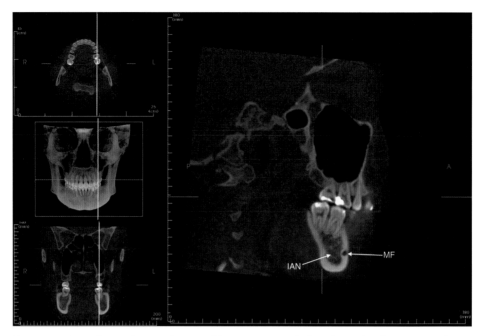

Figure 9.9. Sagittal view showing the mental foramen (MF) with the inferior alveolar nerve canal (IAN) posterior to it. Yellow line showing sagittal plane on left views (axial, 3D reconstruction, and coronal).

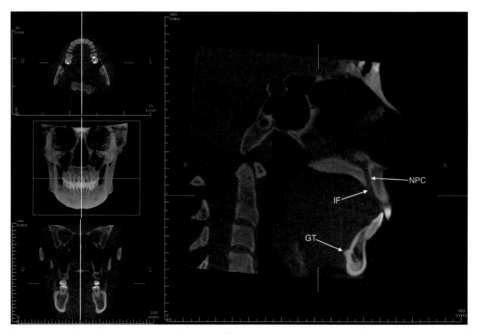

Figure 9.10. Sagittal view showing the nasopalatine canal (NPC), incisive foramen (IF), and genial tubercle (GT). Yellow line showing sagittal plane on left views (axial, 3D reconstruction, and coronal).

Anatomic Variants/Developmental Anomalies

Idiopathic Osteosclerosis (Enostosis, Dense Bone Island)

Definition/Clinical Characteristics

A localized idiopathic bone hyperplasia (variant of normal bone trabeculation). This typically develops at a young age and may grow during this period. It is stable in size in adults. This is an asymptomatic finding.

Radiographic Findings

This presents most commonly in the mandibular premolar/molar region. It appears as a well-defined, radiopaque area continuous with the surrounding bone trabeculation (Figures 9.11 and 9.12). The radiopacity is that of cortical bone (Figure 9.13). It may be single or multiple. It is visualized equally on all three views (axial, coronal, and sagittal).

Differential Interpretation

If centered around the apex of a tooth, apical sclerosing osteitis should be considered. Evaluate tooth for vitality or source of inflammation. If multiple areas (5+) are visualized, an underlying systemic condition such as Gardner's syndrome should be considered.

Treatment/Recommendations

No further imaging or treatment is recommended. May be of concern with implant placement.

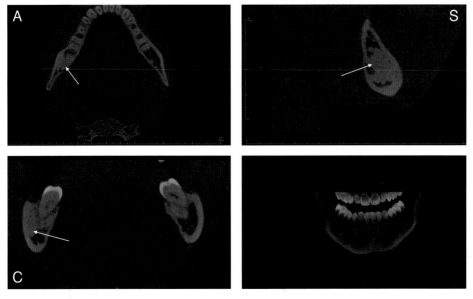

Figure 9.11.   Axial (A), coronal (C), and sagittal (S) views showing a well-defined, radiopaque area (radiopacity of cortical bone) around the roots of the mandibular right second molar (white arrows) consistent with idiopathic osteosclerosis.

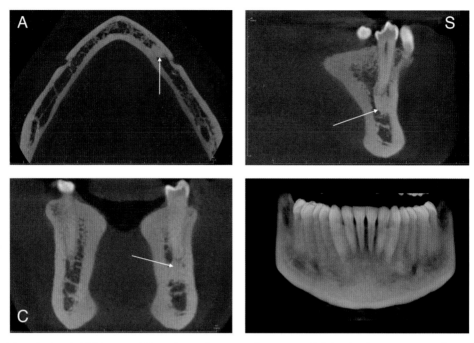

Figure 9.12.   Axial (A), coronal (C), and sagittal (S) views showing a well-defined, radiopaque area (radiopacity of cortical bone) at the apex of the mandibular left first premolar (white arrows) consistent with idiopathic osteosclerosis.

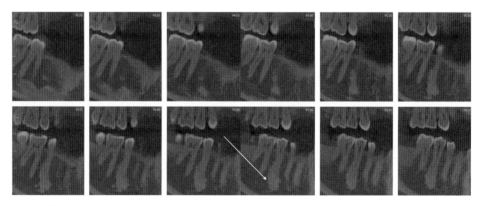

Figure 9.13.   Rotated sagittal views showing a well-defined, radiopaque area (radiopacity of cortical bone) at the apex of a mandibular second premolar (white arrow) consistent with idiopathic osteosclerosis.

Stafne Defect (Mandibular Salivary Gland Defect)

Definition/Clinical Characteristics

A depression on the lingual surface of the mandible typically filled with salivary gland tissue. This is most commonly associated with the submandibular salivary gland. This is an asymptomatic finding. It may grow slowly over time. This is most commonly discovered in the fifth to sixth decade. There is a male predilection.

Radiographic Findings

This presents inferior to the inferior alveolar nerve canal. It appears as a well-defined, round/ovoid, corticated indentation on the lingual surface of the mandible (Figures 9.14–9.16). It may be unilateral or bilateral. It is visualized equally on all three views (axial, coronal, and sagittal).

Differential Interpretation

There is no differential interpretation due to the location and appearance of this finding.

Treatment/Recommendations

Monitoring with radiographs recommended. No further treatment is recommended.

Pathosis

Apical Rarefying Osteitis (Apical Periodontitis)

Definition/Clinical Characteristics

Rarefying osteitis is the loss of bone due to inflammation. It presents at the apex/apices of a tooth/teeth with odontogenic inflammation. Histopathologically, it represents an abscess, cyst, and/or granuloma. There is a wide range of symptoms from asymptomatic to pain, percussion tenderness, and swelling associated with the affected tooth.

Radiographic Findings

This presents centered at the apex of a non-vital tooth. It appears as a well-defined, round/ovoid, radiolucent area with loss of lamina dura of the affected tooth (Figures 9.17 and 9.18). In some cases, a sinus tract may develop (Figure 9.19). In the case of larger lesions, resorption of adjacent teeth/anatomy may occur. In the case of a granuloma, resorption of the associated tooth may occur. It may be single or affect multiple teeth. It is visualized equally on all three views (axial, coronal, and sagittal).

(a)   (b)

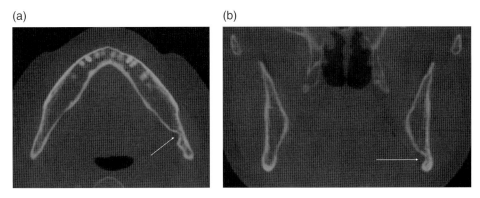

Figure 9.14.   (a) Axial view showing a corticated lingual indentation consistent with a Stafne defect (white arrow). (b) Coronal view showing a corticated lingual indentation consistent with a Stafne defect (white arrow).

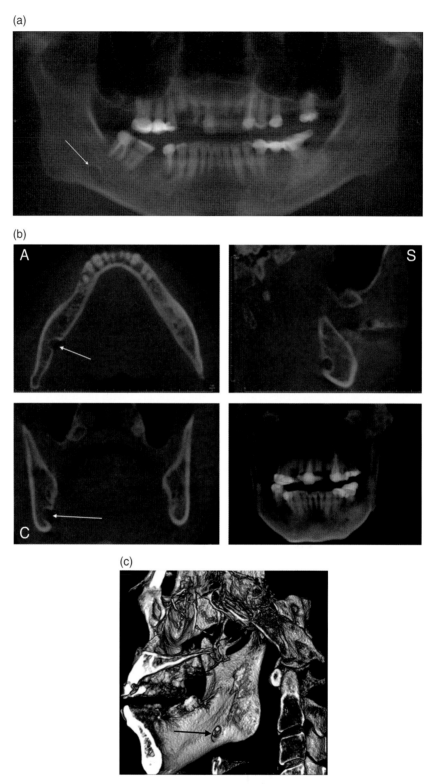

Figure 9.15. (a) Reconstructed pantomograph from a CBCT scan showing a well-defined, corticated, ovoid area (white arrow) inferior to the inferior alveolar nerve canal. (b) Axial (A), coronal (C), and sagittal (S) views showing a Stafne defect as a corticated lingual indentation (white arrows). (c) Reconstructed 3D view showing a Stafne defect as a lingual indentation in the mandible (black arrow).

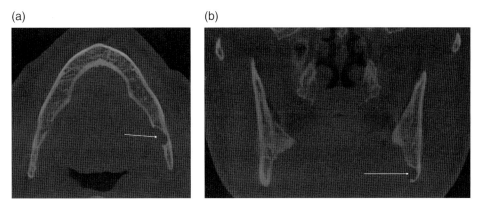

Figure 9.16. (a) Axial view showing a corticated lingual indentation consistent with a Stafne defect (white arrow). (b) Coronal view showing a corticated lingual indentation consistent with a Stafne defect (white arrow).

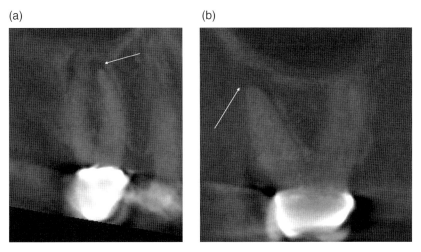

Figure 9.17. (a) Sagittal view showing a well-defined, round radiolucent area (white arrow) at the mesio-buccal root apex of a maxillary molar consistent with apical rarefying osteitis. (b) Coronal view showing a well-defined, radiolucent area (white arrow) at the palatal apex of a maxillary molar with a discontinuity of the palatal cortical plate consistent with apical rarefying osteitis.

Differential Interpretation

Periapical cemento-osseous dysplasia Stage 1 appears similarly but is associated with a vital tooth and will change to a mixed radiopaque/radiolucent appearance over time.

Treatment/Recommendations

Tooth vitality testing is recommended. If the tooth is non-vital, treatment options include endodontic therapy or extraction.

Apical Sclerosing Osteitis

Definition/Clinical Characteristics

Sclerosing osteitis is an inflammatory reaction resulting in deposition of bone surrounding a source of inflammation. It presents at the apex/apices of a tooth/teeth with odontogenic inflammation. This may present in conjunction with apical rarefying

(a)   (b)

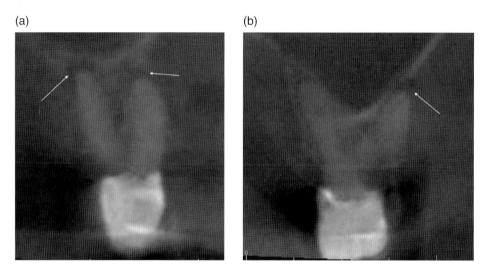

Figure 9.18. (a) Sagittal view showing well-defined, radiolucent areas (white arrows) at the buccal apices of a maxillary molar consistent with apical rarefying osteitis. (b) Coronal view showing a well-defined, radiolucent area (white arrow) at the buccal apex of a maxillary molar with a discontinuity of the facial cortical plate consistent with apical rarefying osteitis.

osteitis. There is a wide range of symptoms from asymptomatic to pain, percussion tenderness, and swelling associated with the affected tooth.

Radiographic Findings

This presents centered around a localized source of inflammation (typically an apex of a tooth). It appears as a diffuse radiopaque area (Figure 9.20). The radiopacity is that of cancellous bone. This may present with apical rarefying osteitis. This may be single or in multiple areas. It is visualized equally on all three views (axial, coronal, and sagittal).

Differential Interpretation

Idiopathic osteosclerosis is a bone hyperplasia that may also present at the apex of a tooth. It will not appear to radiate from the apex (source of inflammation). The radiopacity is that of cortical bone.

Treatment/Recommendations

Recommend evaluation for source of inflammation.

Osteomyelitis

Definition/Clinical Characteristics

A generalized bacterial inflammation of a bone. The most common area in the jaws is the posterior mandible. Patients may present with pain, swelling, and drainage in the affected area. Chronic cases may have intermittent symptomatic periods. This affects all ages with a male predilection.

(a)

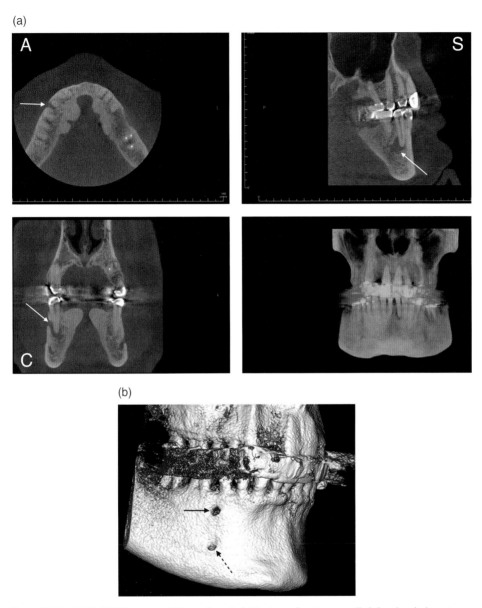

(b)

Figure 9.19. (a) Axial (A), coronal (C), and sagittal (S) views showing a well-defined radiolucent area (white arrows) at the apex of the mandibular right second premolar with a sinus tract opening on the facial surface of the mandible. The appearance is consistent with apical rarefying osteitis. (b) 3D reconstruction showing the sinus tract opening (black arrow) on the facial surface of the mandible superior to the mental foramen (black dashed arrow).

Radiographic Findings

There is a range of bony changes based on the length of inflammation. Acute infections present as an ill-defined loss of bone. Chronic infections present as diffuse bony sclerosis with areas of ill-defined loss of bone (Figure 9.21).

Two radiographic findings seen with osteomyelitis are periostitis and sequestrum.

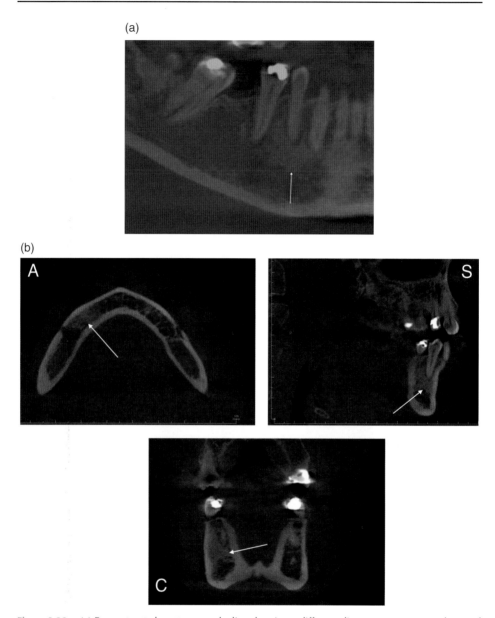

Figure 9.20. (a) Reconstructed pantomograph slice showing a diffuse radiopaque area centered around the apex of the mandibular right first premolar (white arrow) consistent with apical sclerosing osteitis. (b) Axial (A), coronal (C), and sagittal (S) views showing diffuse radiopaque area at the apex of the mandibular right first premolar (white arrows) consistent with apical sclerosing osteitis.

Sequestrum is a non-vital bone fragment surrounded by radiolucent area in the affected jaw (Figure 9.22). This is a hallmark radiographic finding for osteomyelitis.

Periostitis (onion-skin appearance) is an inflammatory reaction of the periosteum overlying the cortical border resulting in layers of new bone formation at the cortical border (Figure 9.23). This presents as layers of radiopacity and radiolucency and is more commonly seen in younger patients.

(a)

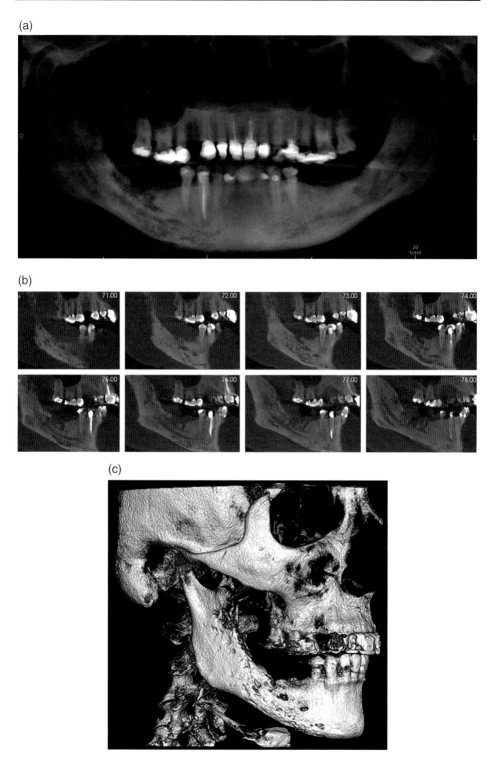

(b)

(c)

Figure 9.21.   (a) Reconstructed pantomograph showing irregular bone loss and sclerosis in the posterior right mandible consistent with osteomyelitis. (b) Rotated sagittal views showing irregular bone destruction with sclerosis in the posterior right mandible consistent with osteomyelitis. (c) 3D reconstruction showing bone destruction of the facial cortical plate in the posterior right mandible consistent with osteomyelitis.

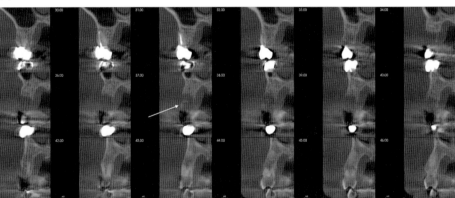

Figure 9.22. (a) Rotated axial (A), coronal (C), and sagittal (S) views showing a separated bone fragment (white arrows) in the posterior right maxilla consistent with a sequestrum. (b) Cross-sectional slices of the right posterior maxilla showing bone loss with a separated bone fragment (white arrow) consistent with a sequestrum.

Differential Interpretation

Fibrous dysplasia has a similar appearance in younger patients. The difference is how the bone enlarges. Periostitis enlarges on the outside of the cortical border, whereas fibrous dysplasia enlarges from inside the cortical borders and may cause thinning of the cortical border.

(a)

(b)

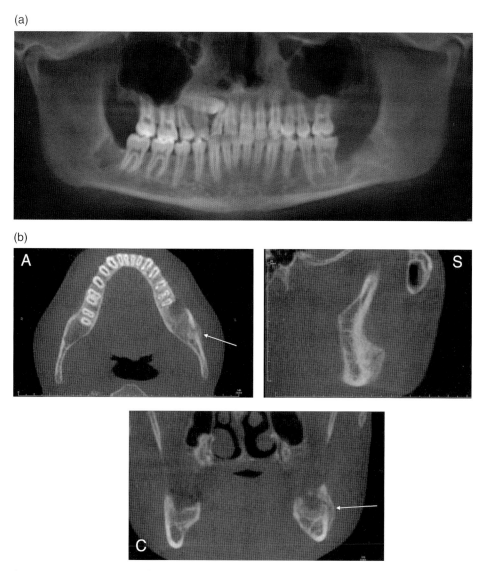

Figure 9.23. (a) Reconstructed pantomograph showing irregular bone loss in the posterior left mandible. (b) Axial (A), coronal (C), and sagittal (S) views showing new bone formation (white arrows) on the external surface of the left mandible consistent with periostitis.

Malignancy may also present as an ill-defined loss of bone without any inflammatory reaction (periostitis).

Paget's disease of bone presents with diffuse bone sclerosis, but this will affect the entire bone.

Both osteoradionecrosis and bisphosphonate-related osteonecrosis have similar radiographic appearances, and the patient's history will need to be determined for either a history of radiation therapy or bisphosphonate therapy.

Treatment/Recommendations

Referral for further treatment/biopsy of the area.

Incidental Findings

Cemento-Osseous Dysplasia

Definition/Clinical Characteristics

Cemento-osseous dysplasia is a lesion composed of abnormal bone and cementum-like components at the apices of vital teeth. Based on the location and extent of the disease, different classifications are given. Periapical cemento-osseous dysplasia refers to localized findings in the anterior mandible. Florid cemento-osseous is when two or four quadrants are affected. It is typically asymptomatic. This is more common in blacks and Asians. There is a female predilection with a mean age of 39.

Radiographic Findings

This presents as a well-defined area at the apex/apices of teeth. There are three radiographic stages of the internal structure of this finding progressing from stage 1 to stage 3 over time. Stage 1 presents as purely radiolucent. Stage 2 presents as mixed radiopaque/radiolucent (Figures 9.24–9.26). Stage 3 presents as purely radiopaque. The associated teeth are vital. It is visualized equally on all three views (axial, coronal, and sagittal).

Differential Interpretation

Stage 1: Apical rarefying osteitis also presents as a well-defined radiolucent area at the apex of a tooth. It is important to test tooth vitality as this is associated with a non-vital tooth.

Stage 2: Cemento-ossifying fibroma is a mixed radiopaque/radiolucent area more commonly seen in the mandibular premolar region. This will not progress to a purely radiopaque stage over time.

Stage 3: Cementoblastoma may present as a well-defined radiopaque area but is more common in mandibular molars, and it will be attached to the tooth root.

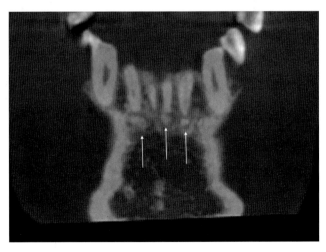

Figure 9.24.   Coronal view showing multiple well-defined, mixed radiopaque/radiolucent areas at the apices of the mandibular incisors (white arrows) consistent with periapical cemento-osseous dysplasia.

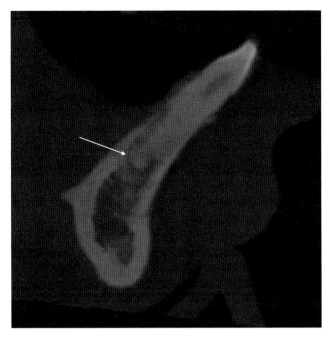

Figure 9.25. Sagittal view showing a well-defined, mixed radiopaque/radiolucent area at the apex of a mandibular incisor (white arrow) consistent with periapical cemento-osseous dysplasia.

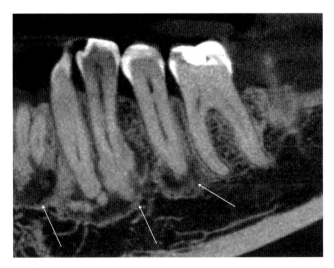

Figure 9.26. Reconstructed pantomograph slice from a quadrant scan showing multiple well-defined, mixed radiopaque/radiolucent areas (white arrows) in the left mandible consistent with florid cemento-osseous dysplasia.

Treatment/Recommendations

No treatment necessary. If stage 1 (purely radiolucent) seen, tooth vitality testing recommended. Recommend monitoring to evaluate radiographic changes through stages.

Odontoma

Definition/Clinical Characteristics

An odontoma is a tumor composed of enamel, dentin, cementum, and pulp tissue. This is the most common odontogenic tumor. These components may present as an irregular mass (complex) versus tooth-like entities (compound). Compound odontomas are more common than complex odontomas. They are frequently associated with delayed eruption of a tooth. There is no sex predilection.

(a)

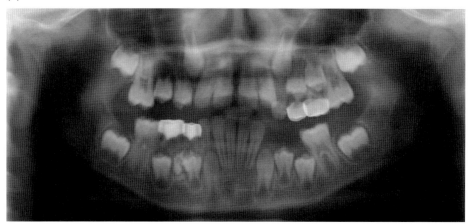

(b)

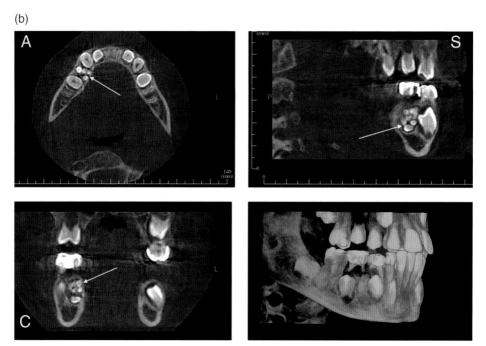

Figure 9.27.　(a) 2D pantomograph showing a well-defined, mixed radiopaque/radiolucent area between the developing right mandibular premolars. There are multiple well-defined, tooth-like structures in this area. The appearance is consistent with a compound odontoma. (b) Axial (A), coronal (C), and sagittal (S) views showing multiple small tooth-like structures (white arrows) in a single follicle in the right posterior mandible consistent with a compound odontoma.

Radiographic Findings

Compound: These are most commonly found in the anterior maxilla. They present as a well-defined, corticated mixed radiopaque/radiolucent area. The radiopaque components appear as small tooth-like structures all within a single follicle (Figures 9.27 and 9.28). It is typically single. It is visualized equally on all three views (axial, coronal, and sagittal).

Complex: These are most commonly found in the mandibular molar region. They present as a well-defined, corticated mixed radiopaque/radiolucent area. The radiopaque aspects have the radiopacity of tooth structure but no defined shape. It is typically single. It is visualized equally on all three views (axial, coronal, and sagittal).

Differential Interpretation

There is no differential interpretation for a compound odontoma due to appearance of multiple tooth-like structures. A cemento-ossifying fibroma should be considered with complex odontomas. Complex odontomas occur in a younger population versus cemento-ossifying fibromas.

Treatment/Recommendations

If the odontoma is interfering with eruption of adjacent teeth, surgical excision may be recommended. If the odontoma is not interfering with adjacent teeth, monitoring is recommended.

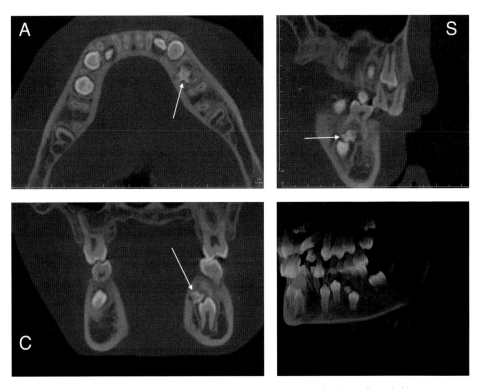

Figure 9.28. Axial (A), coronal (C), and sagittal (S) views showing multiple small tooth-like structures in a single follicle (white arrows) in the left posterior mandible consistent with a compound odontoma.

References

Anatomic Variants/Developmental Anomalies

Asgary, S., and Emadi, N. (2020) Cone-beam computed tomography analysis of lingual mandibular bone depression in the premolar region: a case report. *Clin Case Rep*, 8, 523–6.

Koenig, L. (Ed.). (2012). *Diagnostic Imaging: Oral and Maxillofacial Radiology*. Amirsys.

Mallaya, S., and Lam, E. (Ed.). (2019). *White and Pharaoh's Oral Radiology: Principles and Interpretation*. Mosby.

Pathosis

Dief, S., Veitz-Keenan, A., Amintavakoli, N., et. al (2019). A systematic review on incidental findings in cone beam computed tomography (CBCT) scans. *Dentomaxillofac Radiology*, 48, 20181396.

Koenig, L. (Ed.). (2012). *Diagnostic Imaging: Oral and Maxillofacial Radiology*. Amirsys.

Mallaya, S., and Lam, E. (Ed.). (2019). *White and Pharaoh's Oral Radiology: Principles and Interpretation*. Mosby.

Posadzy, M., Desimpel, J., Vanhoenacker, F. (2018). Cone beam CT of the musculoskeletal system: clinical applications. *Insights Imaging*, 9, 35-45.

Incidental Findings/Other

Koenig, L. (Ed.). (2012). *Diagnostic Imaging: Oral and Maxillofacial Radiology*. Amirsys.

Mallaya, S., and Lam, E. (Ed.). (2019). *White and Pharaoh's Oral Radiology: Principles and Interpretation*. Mosby.

Pereira Cavalcanti, P. H., Leandro Nascimento, E. H., dos Anjos Pontual, M. L., et. al. (2018). Cemento-osseous dysplasias: imaging features based on cone beam computed tomography scans. *Braz Dent J*, 29 (1), 99–104.

Temporomandibular Joints

Gayle Tieszen Reardon

Introduction

Imaging assessments of the temporomandibular joint (TMJ) graphically depict clinically suspected disorders of the jaw joints. It is radiographic examination and imaging that play an important role in the diagnosis and management of most TMJ disorders. Several techniques have been used for the examination of the TMJ, including conventional tomography, magnetic resonance imaging (MRI), arthrography, computed tomography (CT), and, recently, cone beam computed tomography (CBCT). CT and MRI allow for better appreciation of the soft tissues of the joints, which, in turn, allows a better understanding of anatomy and pathophysiology of internal derangements related to disc displacement.

Normal Anatomy and Function

The mandible and temporal bones comprise the osseous components of the TMJ. The head of the mandibular condyle comprises the inferior component of the joint and the temporal bone contributes the mandibular fossa (glenoid fossa) and articular tubercle, forming the superior osseous part of the joint (Figures 10.1–10.4). The articulating surfaces of the TMJs are covered by a thin layer of dense fibrous tissue, rather than the cartilaginous coverings found in most other joints of the body.

The TMJ disc is a biconcave (bowtie-shaped) fibrous structure located between the condylar head and the mandibular fossa of the temporal bone. The disc is round or oval in shape and has a thick periphery and thin dentral portion. Mediolaterally, the disc measures approximately 20 mm. In a normal joint, the posterior band is located over the condyle and the thinner central zone is located between the condyle and the posterior part of the articular tubercle. The anterior band is located under

Interpretation Basics of Cone Beam Computed Tomography, Second Edition.
Edited by Shawneen M. Gonzalez.
© 2021 John Wiley & Sons, Inc. Published 2021 by John Wiley & Sons, Inc.
Companion website: www.wiley.com/go/gonzalez/interpretation

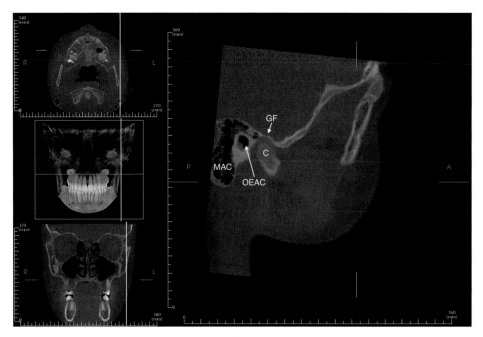

Figure 10.1. Sagittal view showing the glenoid fossa (GF), mandibular condyle (C), osseous external auditory canal (OEAC), and mastoid air cells (MAC). Yellow line showing sagittal plane on left views (axial, 3D reconstruction, and coronal).

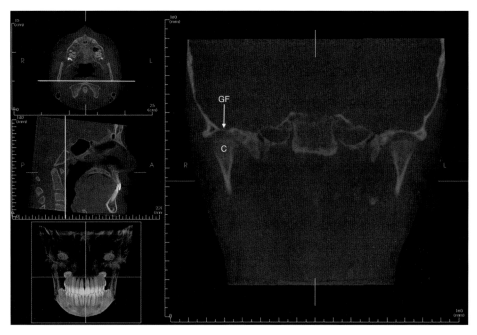

Figure 10.2. Coronal view showing the glenoid fossa (GF) and mandibular condyle (C). Yellow line showing coronal plane on left views (axial and sagittal).

the articular tubercle. The entire joint is surrounded by a joint capsule emerging from the temporal bone and extending to attach to the neck of the condyle. Posteriorly, the disc is attached to the temporal bone and to the condyle by the posterior disc attachment. The posterior attachment is very important in internal

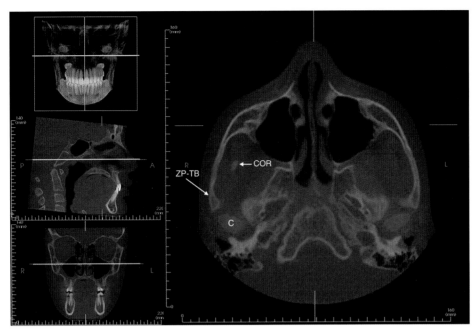

Figure 10.3. Axial view showing the zygomatic process of the temporal bone (ZP-TB), mandibular condyle (C), and coronoid process (COR). Yellow line showing axial level on left views (3D reconstruction, sagittal, and coronal).

derangements of the TMJ. The posterior attachment is also referred to as the bilaminar zone (from old histologic studies), or the retrodiscal tissue, and it consists of loose fibrous connective and elastic tissue components. Anteriorly, the disc attaches to the joint capsule and merges with the superior head of the lateral pterygoid muscle.

The craniomandibular articulation is complex because it involves two separate synovial joints, which function in unison within the same joint capsule. This allows for proportionally greater movement of the TMJ in relation to the actual physical size of the joint. The principal function of the disc is to permit relatively large movements within a small joint while maintaining stability. Rotation and translation occur in both the superior and inferior joint spaces; however, rotation is more evident in the inferior joint space while translation is predominant in the superior joint space. After the initial rotation, translation occurs in the superior and subsequently in the inferior joint space. During translation, the condyle and the disc translate together under the articular tubercle. All during mandibular movement, the thin central portion of the disc is located between the condylar head and the articular tubercle, suggesting that the thicker periphery of the disc and the thick posterior and anterior bands act as functional guide for joint movement.

A fibrous capsule defines the anatomical and functional boundaries of the joint. Medially and laterally, the capsule is firm, which contributes to its stabilization during movement. The medial capsule is not as strong as the lateral capsule, which is reinforced by the temporomandibular ligament laterally. Anteriorly and posteriorly, the capsule is loose enough to allow for mandibular movement. The TMJ is supported by two accessory ligaments to protect the joint during wide excursive movements.

The first is the stylomandibular ligament, which runs from the tip of the styloid process to the angle and posterior border of the mandible. The second, the sphenomandibular ligament, runs from the greater wing of the sphenoid bone to the lingual of the mandibular ramus. The sphenomandibular ligament attaches separately from the medial capsule.

(a)   (b)

(c)   (d)

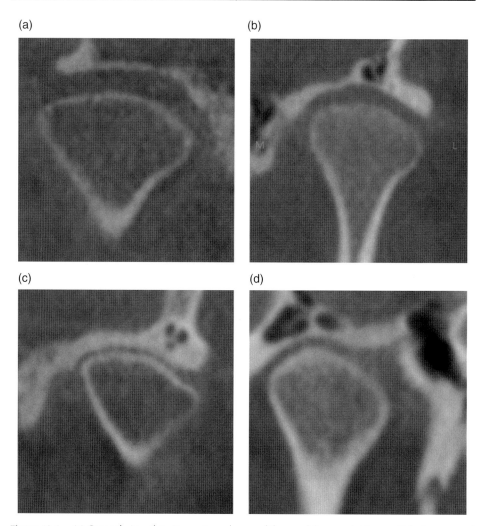

Figure 10.4. (a) Coronal view showing various shapes of the condyle acceptable as within the range of normal. (b) Coronal view showing various shapes of the condyle acceptable as within the range of normal. (c) Coronal view showing various shapes of the condyle acceptable as within the range of normal. (d) Coronal view showing various shapes of the condyle acceptable as within the range of normal.

The capsule encloses the condyle and merges into the periosteum of the condylar neck. Laterally, the firmer attachment of the capsule extends below the condylar neck. It is shorter medially where it blends into the periosteum of the condylar neck below the medial pole of the condyle. The articular capsule completely surrounds the articular surfaces of the concave mandibular fossa (glenoid fossa) and the convex articular eminence, both formed by the squamous part of the temporal bone. Any condyle excursion beyond the anteriosuperior insertion of the capsule is classified as hypermobility.

The capsule consists of two layers, an outer fibrous layer and an inner layer of synovial tissue. The synovial layer produces synovial fluid with a function that serves three purposes: to reduce friction between articular surfaces by serving as a lubricant, to provide nutrition to the nonvascularized tissues of the articulating surfaces and the disc, and to remove debris from the joint spaces. There is only enough synovial fluid to outline the joint surfaces. If larger amounts of joint fluid are present, it is an indication of joint pathology.

The joint has an intracapsular disc that divides the synovial cavity into noncommunicating upper and lower compartments. The disc consists of dense collagenous tissue without innervations or vascularization. In the child and adolescent, the disc is composed of dense collagenous fibers; in the elderly person, it is fibrocartilage. In the newborn, the entire disc is of equal thickness. This changes as the TMJ begins to function. With function, the disc adapts to the configurations of the opposing surfaces, resulting in its final biconcave "bowtie" appearance. The posterior and anterior thick parts are called posterior and anterior bands. The undersurface of the disc and the superior aspect of the condylar head fit perfectly together during all jaw movements.

The disc attaches firmly to the condyle medially and laterally so it is able to move only slightly in the mediolateral direction. Posteriorly, the disc is continuous with the posterior disc attachments (the retrodiscal pad), which consists of loose connective tissue with large elastic fibers and fat. It is highly vascular and well innervated in addition to being outlined by synovial membrane. The posterior attachments can easily become compressed and, because of its structure, it is unfit for articulation, which may occur when the disc is displaced. If the undersurface of the posterior discal attachment is damaged, the disc can translate to a position anterior to the condyle, resulting in an anterior disc displacement.

During jaw movement, the condyle rotates smoothly against the central underside of the disc. The disc and condyle move as an integrated complex in the healthy joint. It is MRI that enables the depiction of both soft and hard tissues of the joint and provides us with visualization of the relationship of the hard and soft tissues.

Developmental Abnormalities

Based on their etiology and time of appearance, developmental conditions can be classified as congenital malformations with associated growth disorders and as primary growth disorders. Hemifacial microsomia, condylar aplasia, condylar hypoplasia, or condylar hyperplasia are the most common craniofacial malformations. Facial asymmetry is the most prevalent clinical sign of developmental conditions in the TMJ region. CBCT and 3D CBCT provide diagnostic information about the size, shape, and accurate position of the mandibular condyle. They also provide information about morphology, inclination, displacement, or deviation of the lateral and medial surfaces of the mandibular rami and body.

Hemifacial Microsomia

Definition/Clinical Characteristics

Hemifacial microsomia is the second most common facial birth defect after cleft palate/lip, occurring in approximately 1 in 5000 live births with variable frequencies reported. It occurs more frequently in males than females. It is the most frequent syndrome from first and second branchial arches. It may not be appreciable in infancy and is usually evident by the age of 4 years. Characteristic clinical findings include facial asymmetry and ear anomalies. The right-side facial underdevelopment is more frequent than left-side underdevelopment. Skin tags between ear and corner of mouth occur. Seventh cranial nerve palsy is frequent. Other findings include dental malocclusion, hypodontia, and plagiocephaly in 10%. Bifacial microsomia has been reported.

It is seen on radiographs as an underdeveloped mandible without a mandibular condyle. A flat zygomatic arch without a mandibular fossa may be evident.

Condylar Aplasia

Condylar aplasia is the absence of one or both condyles.

Condylar Hypoplasia

Definition/Clinical Characteristics/Radiographic Description

Condylar hypoplasia is an undersized condyle with normal morphology. It may be congenital, developmental, or acquired. Some examples include micrognathia, Treacher Collins syndrome, secondary effects of radiation, or the result of infection. It generally presents with an underdeveloped ramus and body of the mandible on the same side, creating asymmetry of the mandible. Degenerative joint disease (DJD) or osteoarthrosis is a long-term sequela (Figures 10.5 and 10.6).

Differential Interpretation

Juvenile rheumatoid arthritis presents with problems in other joints or the result of Rh factor incompatibility. Another differential includes severe DJD; however, this is found in an older-aged individual.

Treatment/Recommendations

Treatment options include orthognathic surgery, bone grafts, and orthodontic therapy.

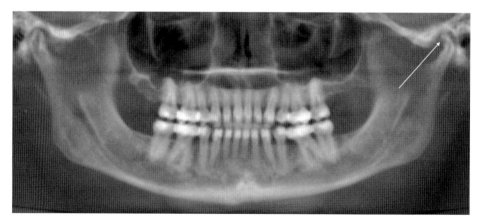

Figure 10.5.   Reconstructed pantomograph from a CBCT scan showing left condylar hypoplasia (white arrow).

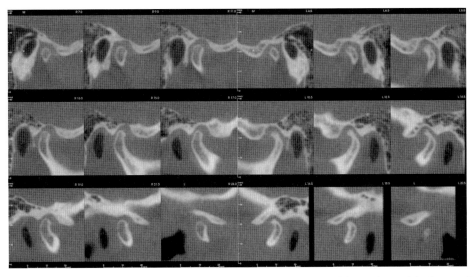

Figure 10.6.   Rotated sagittal cross-sectional slices of the right and left condyles. Right condyle shape and size within the range of normal. Left condyle is smaller than the range of normal.

Condylar Hyperplasia

Definition/Clinical Characteristics/Radiographic Description

Condylar hyperplasia is the enlargement and occasional deformity of the mandibular condyle. There is an increase in cortical thickness with maintenance of a normal trabecular pattern. This is most commonly seen in young males with a mean age of 20 years. It presents as hyperplasia of the ipsilateral mandible in the same side as the condylar hyperplasia and mandibular asymmetry. It is generally self-limiting and ends at approximately the same time as cessation of skeletal growth (Figures 10.7 and 10.8).

Differential Interpretation

Differential interpretation includes osteochondroma, condylar osteoma, and large osteophyte or beaking of the mandibular condyle. Osteochondroma is irregular growth, which continues after the cessation of skeletal growth. Large osteophyte or beaking of the mandibular condyle are characteristic of osteoarthrosis and are found in older-aged individuals.

Treatment/Recommendations

Treatment is frequently orthodontics with orthognathic surgery.

Juvenile Arthrosis (Boering's Arthrosis)

Definition/Clinical Characteristics/Radiographic Description

Juvenile arthrosis presenting with condylar hypoplasia: Initially the condyle presents within the range of normal and becomes abnormal during growth. It presents with secondary degenerative changes and is typically seen in females. A "toadstool appearance" with marked flattening and apparent elongation of the superior surface and

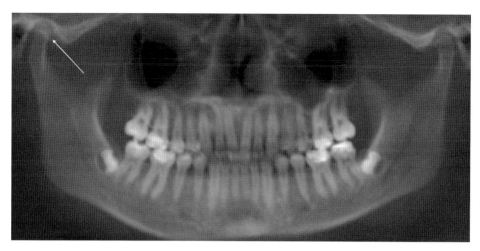

Figure 10.7. Reconstructed pantomograph from a CBCT scan showing right condylar hyperplasia (white arrow).

(a)   (b)

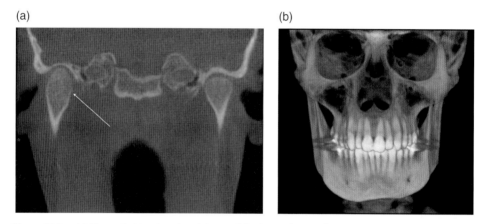

Figure 10.8. (a) Coronal view showing right condylar hyperplasia (white arrow). (b) 3D reconstruction showing mandibular asymmetry.

posterior inclination of the mandibular condyle is frequently seen. The condylar neck is short or may be absent. There is flattening of the mandibular (glenoid) fossa and deepening of antegonial notch(es).

Differential Interpretation

Differential interpretation includes developmental condylar hypoplasia, rheumatoid arthritis, DJD, and condylar degeneration after orthognathic or TMJ surgery.

Treatment/Recommendations

Orthognathic surgery and/or orthodontics.

Coronoid Hyperplasia

Definition/Clinical Characteristics/Radiographic Description

Coronoid hyperplasia may be developmental or acquired. It may be secondary to ankylosis. It is generally seen in males around the time of puberty and presents with a progressive inability to open their mouth. The coronoid process is considered hyperplastic if the tip of the coronoid process extends at least 1 cm above the inferior rim of the zygomatic arch. It may cause remodeling of the zygomatic process of maxilla.

Differential Interpretation

Differential interpretation includes an osteochondroma or osteoma due to its irregular shape, which may develop secondary to other causes of trismus. Example: soft-tissue causes or TMJ ankylosis.

Treatment/Recommendations

Surgical removal with postoperative physiotherapy.

Bifid Condyle

Definition/Clinical Characteristics/Radiographic Description

The condyle presents with a vertical depression, notch, or deep cleft in the condylar head. The location of the "notch" may be in the mediolateral or anteroposterior plane (Figures 10.9–10.11).

(a)   (b)

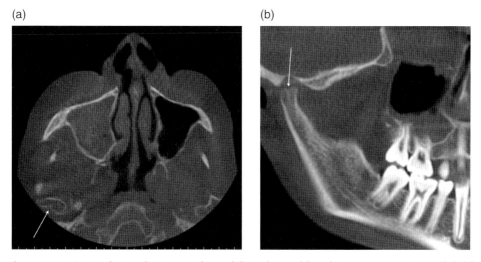

Figure 10.9. (a) Axial view showing notching of the right condyle (white arrow) consistent with bifid condyle. (b) Rotated sagittal view showing notching on the superior aspect of the condyle (white arrow) consistent with a bifid condyle.

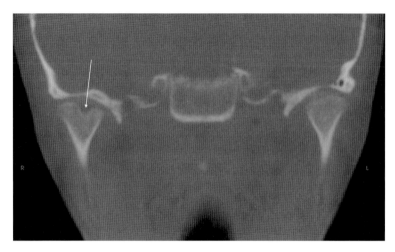

Figure 10.10. Coronal view showing notching on superior aspect of right condyle (white arrow) consistent with bifid condyle.

Differential Interpretation

A vertical fracture may appear like a bifid condyle and may also be an etiology for bifid condyle.

Treatment/Recommendations

Treatment is indicated only if the patient is symptomatic.

Soft-Tissue Abnormalities

Internal Derangements

Internal derangement is a general orthopedic term implying a mechanical fault that interferes with the smooth action of a joint. Internal derangement is thus a functional diagnosis. For the TMJ, the most common internal derangement is disc displacement. This is most often the disc displaced anteriorly, anterolaterally, or anteromedially. When this occurs, the posterior band of the disc prolapses anteriorly rather than remaining in its normal position between the condylar head and mandibular fossa. This results in positioning of the condyle beneath the posterior disc attachment rather than under the disc, causing the condyle to close on the posterior attachment (retrodiscal tissues) rather than upon the disc itself.

Medial or lateral displacements of the disc are also relatively common. Posterior disc displacement also occurs but rarely. When posterior disc displacement occurs, it is seen in conjunction with medial disc displacement. Pure lateral and medial disc displacements do occur but not as commonly as those in conjunction with anterior disc displacements.

Functionally, disc displacements occur with and without reduction. In disc displacement with reduction, the disc is anteriorly displaced in the closed-mouth position but reverts to a normal superior position during opening. In disc displacement without reduction, the disc lies anterior to the condyle during all mandibular movements and the normal condyle-disc relationship is not resumed.

(a)

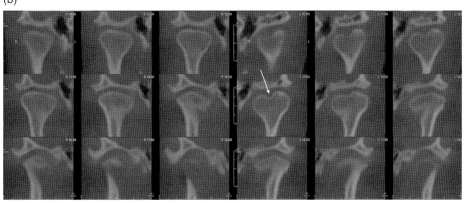

(b)

(c)

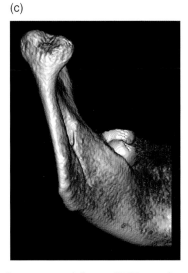

Figure 10.11. (a) Reconstructed pantomograph from a CBCT scan showing superior notching of the left condyle (white arrow) consistent with a bifid condyle. (b) Rotated coronal cross-sectional slices of the right and left condyles with superior notching of the left condyle (white arrow) consistent with a bifid condyle. (c) 3D reconstruction of left condyle showing superior notching consistent with a bifid condyle.

Summary of internal derangement:

■ There is an abnormality in position and morphology of the articular disc, which may interfere with normal function of the joint.
■ Most often the displacement is to the anterior; however, the disc can also be displaced medially and laterally.
■ Causes of disc displacement include parafunctional habits, jaw injuries, whiplash injury, or forced opening beyond the normal range of movement.
■ A "reducing" disc resumes its normal position relative to the position of the condyle; a click is present.
■ A "nonreducing" disc refers to a disc that remains displaced throughout the entire range of mandibular movement and may lead to a closed or open lock. The condyle and disc are never together in their "normal" and desired relationship.
■ Internal derangements may be symptomatic or asymptomatic.

The disc may become deformed, thickened, fibrotic, or perforated.

Remodeling and Arthritis

Remodeling

Definition/Clinical Characteristics/Radiographic Description

Remodeling occurs due to adaptive response to excessive forces applied to the joint. Alterations in the shape of the condyle and articular eminence include flattening, cortical thickening, subchondral sclerosis, or abnormal appearance (only if pain and/or dysfunction present or severe radiographic changes are seen). It may be unilateral and is not invariably a precursor to DJD.

Differential Interpretation

Differential interpretation includes early DJD with erosions, osteophytes, and loss of joint space.

Treatment/Recommendations

There is no treatment necessary. An occlusal splint may be considered.

Degenerative Joint Disease, Osteoarthritis

Definition/Clinical Characteristics

When the ability of the joint to adapt to excessive forces is exceeded, breakdown occurs. Etiology includes acute trauma, hypermobility of the joint, parafunction, and/or internal disc derangement. This is not an inflammatory condition, so "osteoarthritis" is a misnomer. It is more commonly seen in females than males. Deterioration includes the loss of articular cartilage and bone erosion. Proliferation includes cortical thickening, osteophyte formation, sclerosis of the articular surface, and subchondral sclerosis.

Radiographic Description

Radiographically DJD presents with flattening, subchondral sclerosis, loss of cortex/surface erosion, Ely cyst/subchondral cyst formation, and osteophyte, which can form loose joint bodies known as joint mice. There is reduced joint space and long-term nonreducing disc displacement, which can lead to DJD. Anterior open bite can occur if the condyle is resorbed and articular surface of temporal bone is also resorbed (Figures 10.12–10.15).

Differential Interpretation

Differential interpretation is broken into two categories: erosive and proliferative. Radiographic erosive differential includes rheumatoid arthritis with severe erosion. Radiographic proliferative differential includes osteochondroma and osteoma.

Treatment/Recommendations

Treatment is a variety of things including splint therapy, anti-inflammatory drugs, and/or physiotherapy.

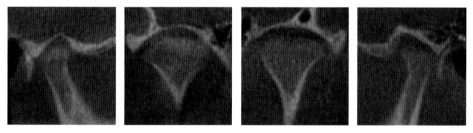

Figure 10.12. Sagittal and coronal slices showing normal condylar morphology.

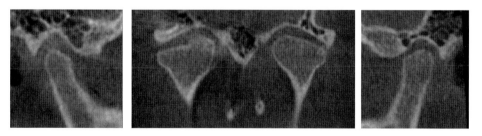

Figure 10.13. Sagittal and coronal slices showing mild flattening consistent with mild DJD changes.

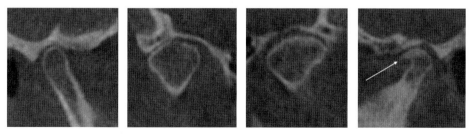

Figure 10.14. Sagittal and coronal slices showing flattening with anterior osteophyte formation (white arrow) of the left condyle consistent with moderate DJD changes.

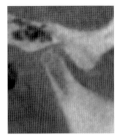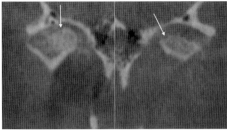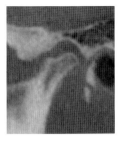

Figure 10.15.   Sagittal and coronal slices showing flattening with loss of cortication (white arrow) consistent with moderate to severe DJD changes.

Osteoarthrosis (Degenerative Arthritis)

Definition/Clinical Characteristics

Osteoarthritis or degenerative arthritis is an age-related disorder that is more frequent in females than in males. The ratio of females to males with this degenerative condition is approximately 7:1. The progression and severity of osseous changes in the condylar head and mandibular fossa tend to increase with age. Patients with osteoarthritis affecting the TMJ usually complain of pain or tenderness in the joint and masticatory muscles, reduced range of motion or deviating jaw function, and crepitus during mandibular movements. CBCT is a valuable imaging modality for the diagnosis of degenerative changes in the osseous components of the TMJ.

Radiographic Description

The most common radiographic findings in early osteoarthritic changes include flattening of the condyle, irregular cortical outlines, cortical bone erosions and subchondral cyst formation, osteophyte formation, reduced joint space, and bony contact with mouth open. In moderate or severe osteoarthritis, osseous changes include extensive osteophyte formation, subcortical cyst formation, resorption of the condylar head or mandibular fossa, absence of joint space, or bony contact and sclerosis of both the condyle and mandibular fossa. Sclerosis is a less-frequent radiographic finding, but it develops secondarily in the more progressive forms of the disease and in older age groups (Figures 10.16–10.18).

Rheumatoid Arthritis

Definition/Clinical Characteristics

Rheumatoid arthritis is the most common chronic inflammatory disease of unknown etiology and is classified as one of the collagen-vascular (autoimmune) diseases. It primarily affects the periarticular structures, such as the synovial membrane capsule, tendon sheaths, and ligaments. Rheumatoid arthritis affects mostly women, with a female to male ratio of 3:1 and a peak onset in patients between 40 and 60 years of age. Patients with rheumatoid arthritis usually complain of bitemporal headache, dull pain worsening with function, and a limitation of condylar movement. An anterior open bite secondary to condylar changes can occur. The clinical examination may reveal pain on palpation, crepitus, and hypomobility. In the early stages, small peripheral joints of the hands and feet are affected first. Clinical and radiologic

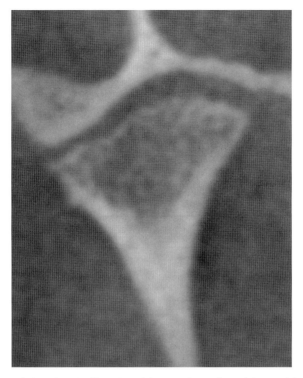

Figure 10.16.   Coronal view showing flattening of the superior surface of the condyle.

examinations reveal involvement of the TMJ in about 70% of patients with rheumatoid arthritis. It is also seen in the knees, hands, and other joints. In late stages of the disease, ankylosis may develop.

Radiographic Description

The most common radiographic findings in the condylar head and mandibular fossa are flattening, erosions, resorption, and sclerosis. In many cases, the joint space may be reduced. In late stages of the disease, radiographic examination may reveal osteophyte formation on the condylar head, a sharp pointed condyle, and posterior ramus shortened in length causing premature posterior occlusion and anterior open bite. Radiographic findings in patients with rheumatoid arthritis are similar to those in patients with osteoarthritis. However, reduced joint space and osteophyte formation are more common in patients with osteoarthritis, whereas erosions and resorption of the condylar head are more frequently found in patients with rheumatoid arthritis (Figures 10.19 and 10.20).

Differential Interpretation

Differential interpretation includes severe DJD and psoriatic arthritis. Psoriatic arthritis patients will have a history of skin lesions, osteopenia, and severe erosions of articular eminence, which are more characteristic of rheumatoid arthritis.

Treatment/Recommendations

Treatment options include analgesics, nonsteroidal anti-inflammatory drugs (NSAIDs), corticosteroids, physiotherapy, and/or joint replacement surgery.

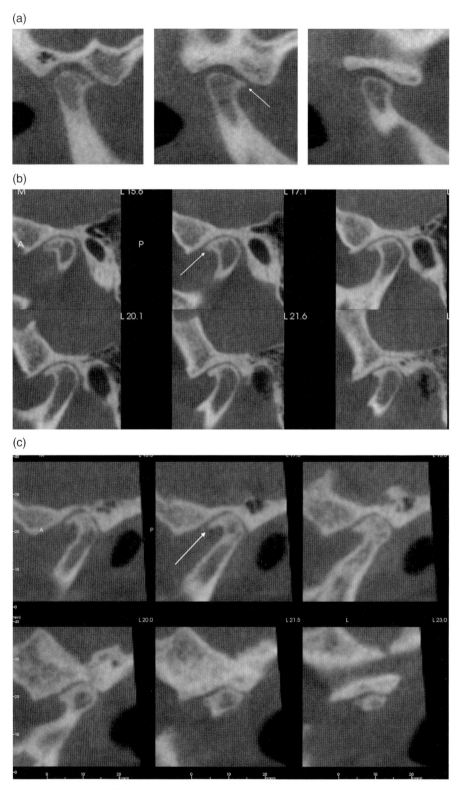

Figure 10.17. (a) Rotated sagittal cross-sectional slices showing anterior osteophyte formation (white arrow). (b) Rotated sagittal cross-sectional slices showing anterior osteophyte formation (white arrow). (c) Rotated sagittal cross-sectional slices showing anterior osteophyte formation (white arrow).

(a)

(b)

(c)

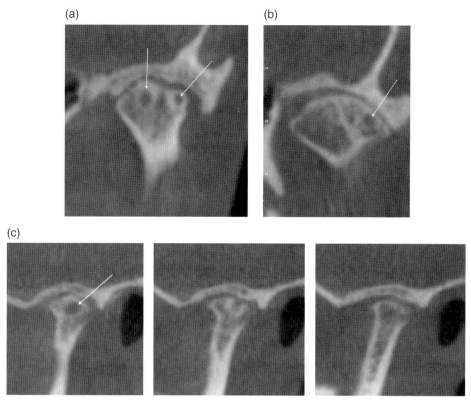

Figure 10.18.   (a) Coronal view showing subchondral cyst formation (white arrows). (b) Coronal view showing subchondral cyst formation (white arrow). (c) Rotated sagittal cross-sectional slices showing subchondral cyst formation (white arrow).

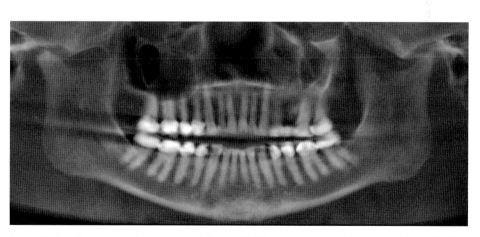

Figure 10.19.   Reconstructed pantomograph from a CBCT scan of patient with rheumatoid arthritis. Note the severe flattening and loss of condylar height bilaterally.

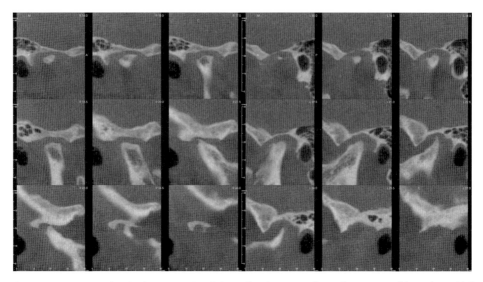

Figure 10.20.   Rotated sagittal cross-sectional slices showing severe bony destruction of the right and left condyles.

Juvenile Arthritis (Juvenile Rheumatoid Arthritis/Juvenile Chronic Arthritis/Still's Disease)

Definition/Clinical Characteristics

Juvenile arthritis is a chronic inflammatory disease typically found in patients less than 16 years of age with a mean age of 5 years. It presents with synovial hypertrophy; joint effusion; and swollen, painful joints. There is cartilage and bone destruction. Rheumatoid factor may be present. Involvement of the TMJ occurs in approximately 40% of all cases. It may be either unilateral or bilateral. Clinical characteristics include micrognathia, which is seen in the young with less development of the mandible, a "bird face," and anterior open bite.

Radiographic Description

Radiographic findings include osteopenia and impaired mandibular growth. Changes in the TMJs include erosions, "pencil-shaped" small condyle, flattening, fibrous ankylosis, secondary degenerative changes, abnormal disc shape, and deepening of the antegonial notch. The ramus may present with diminished height, dorsal bending, or obtuse angle of ramus relative to the body of the mandible (Figures 10.21 and 10.22).

Psoriatic Arthritis

Definition/Clinical Characteristics/Radiographic Description

Psoriatic arthritis has skin lesions present. The TMJs are associated in 7% of all cases. These patients are seronegative, so no rheumatoid factor is present, and it is indistinguishable from rheumatoid arthritis on radiographs. Occasionally, profound sclerotic changes are evident.

(a) (b)

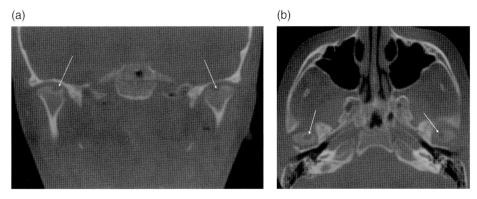

Figure 10.21.   (a) Coronal view showing erosions on the superior aspect of the right and left condyles (white arrows) in a patient with juvenile arthritis. (b) Axial view showing erosions on the superior aspect of the right and left condyles (white arrows) in a patient with juvenile arthritis.

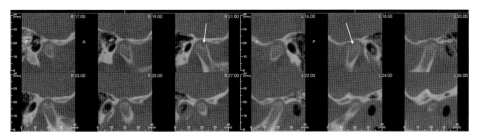

Figure 10.22.   Rotated sagittal cross-sectional slices showing erosions of the right and left condyles (white arrows) in a patient with juvenile arthritis.

Septic Arthritis

Definition/Clinical Characteristics

Septic arthritis is a rare infection and inflammation of a joint. The infection can spread from either the parotid, otic, mastoid, osteomyelitis from mandibular body/ramus, middle ear infection, or hematogenous spread from distant nidus. It is more commonly seen in people with rheumatoid arthritis, diabetes, and/or immunosuppression. Children may present with septic arthritis after blunt trauma with hematoma formation, which is adequate for microorganism growth. It is typically unilateral with the mandible deviated to the unaffected side due to joint effusion.

Radiographic Description

Radiographically the joint space may be widened with erosion and thinning of the cortex. Other radiographic findings include osteopenia, sequestrum formation, periosteal reaction, and osseous ankylosis. Inhibited mandibular growth can take place if it occurs in a young person.

Differential Interpretation

Differential interpretation includes DJD and rheumatoid arthritis. Diagnosis can be made via joint aspirate and is typically unilateral with clinical signs and symptoms of infection. Other inflammatory changes in adjacent areas seen include the mastoid air cells, mandibular ramus, and parotid. On MRI T2 weighted image joint effusion, abscess, and muscle enlargement may be seen. Scintigraphy with technetium 99 shows increased bone metabolism and gallium shows signs of infection.

Synovial Chondromatosis (Synovial Chondrometaplasia, Osteochondromatosis)

Definition/Clinical Characteristics

Synovial chondromatosis is a rare benign condition that mainly affects the superior joint space, although it can involve the inferior joint space when a perforated or a deformed disc is present. It is characterized by the formation of fragments of cartilage and loose bodies in the synovial membrane of the affected joint. Synovial chondromatosis is more frequent in females than males, with a predilection ratio of 4:1, respectively. Clinical symptoms of synovial chondromatosis are not pathognomic and usually include joint swelling, pain, intracapsular sounds (clicking, crepitus, or both), and a limitation of joint movement.

Radiographic Description

The most common CBCT findings in patients with TMJ synovial chondromatosis include the presence of multiple, loose, calcified nodules in the joint space, sclerosis of the mandibular fossa and the condylar head, irregularity of the osseous cortical surface, and often widening of the joint space. Usually, the condyle exhibits osseous changes similar to those seen in osteoarthritis patients. Loose calcified nodules in CBCT images can appear as multiple articular radiopacities of varying sizes and shapes. In many cases, temporal bone sclerosis and extension of the lesion into the intracranial fossa, infratemporal fossa, or lateral pterygoid muscle are seen.

Differential Interpretation

Differential interpretation includes chondrocalcinosis, synovial chondromatosis, DJD with joint mice, and chondro/osteosarcoma. Chondrocalcinosis presents with larger nodules and peripheral cortex than synovial chondromatosis. Synovial chondromatosis has larger loose bodies. Chondro/osteosarcoma present with severe bone destruction.

Treatment

Treatment includes removal of the loose bodies and removal of abnormal synovial tissue.

Chondrocalcinosis (Pseudogout, Calcium Pyrophosphate Dihydrate Deposition Disease)

Definition/Clinical Characteristics

Chondrocalcinosis is an acute or chronic synovitis with precipitation of calcium pyrophosphate dehydrate crystals in joint space. It is uncommon in the TMJ and usually involves other joints. It is more commonly unilateral and more common in males than females.

Radiographic Description

It appears as fine radiopacities with even distribution in joint space as compared to synovial chondromatosis. Bone erosions with severe increase in condylar bone density and swelling and edema of muscles may be present (Figure 10.23).

Differential Interpretation

Differential interpretation includes synovial chondromatosis, DJD with joint mice, and chondro/osteosarcoma.

Treatment

Treatment options include surgical removal of deposits, steroids, aspirin, NSAIDS, and colchicine.

(a)   (b)

(c)

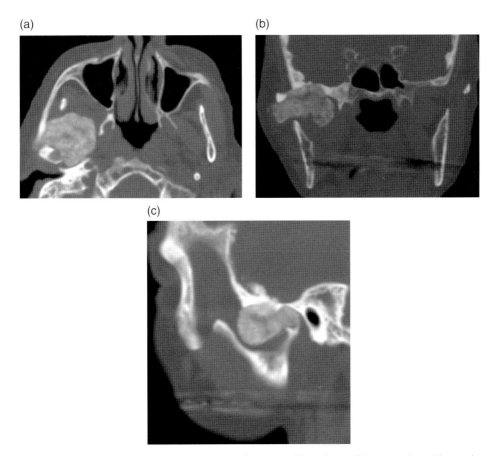

Figure 10.23.   (a) Axial view showing increased radiopacity of the right condyle in a patient with pseudo-gout. (b) Coronal view showing increased radiopacity of the right condyle in a patient with pseudogout. (c) Sagittal view showing increased radiopacity of the right condyle in a patient with pseudogout.

Effusion

Definition/Clinical Characteristics

Effusion is influx of fluid into a joint. It may be either trauma from hemorrhage or inflammation from exudate. Causes include internal derangement, traumatic injuries, arthritis, and rheumatic diseases. Clinical findings include swelling, pain, limited motion, hearing difficulties, and difficulty occluding posterior teeth because of fluid in the joint.

Radiographic Description

T2 weighted MRI shows internal derangement with normal joints and high signal (hyperintense signal).

Differential Interpretation

Septic arthritis with signs and symptoms of infection present in septic arthritis.

Treatment

Treatment options include anti-inflammatories and surgical drainage occasionally.

Dislocation

Definition/Clinical Characteristics

The condyle may present outside the mandibular fossa but inside the capsule. It occurs bilaterally and is most commonly displaced anteriorly. It may be associated with condylar fracture. Clinical findings include inability to close the mouth without pain and/or muscle spasms. It is possible to reduce the mandible by manipulation.

Radiographic Description

The condyles are located anterior and superior to the summit of articular eminence (clinical information is important, because it could be normal range of motion for that specific patient).

Differential Interpretation

Fracture dislocations.

Treatment

Treatment is typically manual manipulation and surgery for fractures.

Fracture

Definition/Clinical Characteristics

The consequences of traumatic injury to the condyle depend on its location. Condylar fractures may be intracapsular or extracapsular. Extracapsular fractures are (subsequently) classified into high, medium, or low with regard to their position. These fractures can be displaced, nondisplaced, or dislocated, and depending on the direction of the fracture, they can be horizontal, vertical, or sagittal. If the fracture is located in the condylar neck, the condylar head often becomes dislocated. CBCT is a useful diagnostic tool for the diagnosis of TMJ fracture.

Radiographic Description

A cortical outline irregularity can be (or is usually) depicted and, in case of a condylar neck fracture, the condylar head is usually dislocated in a forward-medial direction. The most common location is the condylar neck with dislocation of condylar head. Unilateral is more common and may be accompanied by parasymphyseal or body fracture on the opposite side. It can lead to growth inhibition in a young person. For those less than 10 years, there is a high remodeling potential and less deformity than older patients. For those less than 3 years, severe asymmetries are possible. Other radiographic findings include ankylosis, radiolucent or radiopaque lines, step defects, and condylar head fracture with vertical or compressive patterns. Remodeling typically shows as flattening, DJD. Hemarthrosis may present with blood in the joint.

Differential Interpretation

Differential interpretation includes developmental abnormalities. A Towne's view shows medial displacement of condyle.

Treatment

No treatment is necessary if adequate mandibular movement is present.

Neonatal Fractures

Forceps injury during delivery may lead to fracture of condyle(s). Clinically, this presents as severe mandibular hypoplasia, lack of development of the glenoid fossa, and eminence with "partly opened pair of scissors" appearance due to overlapping of fracture fragments. Differential includes developmental hypoplasia. Treatment includes orthodontics and orthognathic surgery for mandibular asymmetry.

Ankylosis

Definition/Clinical Characteristics

True ankylosis is in the joint and may be either fibrous or bony. False ankylosis is unrelated to the joint, and examples include muscle spasm, myositis ossificans, or coronoid process hyperplasia. If it is unilateral, possible causes include trauma or infection. Common causes for bilateral ankylosis include rheumatoid arthritis. If present during infancy, it is likely due to a birth injury caused by forceps.

Radiographic Description

Fibrous ankylosis presents as irregular erosions on articular surfaces with a narrowed joint space and jigsaw puzzle appearance. Bony ankylosis presents as small or large osseous bridges/large bony masses. Other radiographic findings include degenerative changes, coronoid hyperplasia, and deepening of antegonial notch because of the pull of muscles when opening the mouth.

Differential Interpretation

Differential interpretation includes condylar tumor. With a history of trauma, infection, or other joint diseases, should consider ankylosis.

Treatment

Treatment includes surgical removal of osseous bridge or bony mass.

Tumors

Benign Tumors

Definition/Clinical Characteristics

Osteochondroma or osteocartilaginous exostosis is the most common benign tumor of the TMJ and is most commonly seen in the second or third decade of life. It usually affects the condyle and is defined as an exophytic bone mass emanating from the cortex, which may cause limited mouth opening and jaw deviation to the contralateral side. Most frequently, patients with condylar osteochondroma develop facial asymmetry and/or malocclusion. In radiographic examinations, osteochondroma is depicted as a tapering radiopaque mass usually extending from the anteromedial aspect of the condyle along the tendon of the lateral pterygoid. CBCT findings show an enlarged condyle with irregular outline or an abnormal pedunculated mass attached to the condyle.

Benign neoplasms seen in the TMJs include osteochondroma, osteoma, osteoblastoma, chondroblastoma, fibromyxoma, giant cell lesions, aneurysmal bone cysts, and Langerhans cell histiocytosis, which is considered benign in Mallaya and Lam (2019).

Radiographic Description

There is a range of radiographic findings including condylar enlargement, irregular in shape, altered trabecular pattern, radiolucency/radiopacity, or abnormal pedunculated mass.

Differential Interpretation

Unilateral condylar hyperplasia.

Treatment

Surgical excision.

Malignant Tumors

Malignant tumors of the TMJ are very rare lesions. The majority of reported cases in the literature include osteosarcomas, chondrosarcomas, and metastatic tumors. Osteosarcoma and chondrosarcoma are malignancies with a slight male predilection and are characterized by the formation of neoplastic bone or cartilage by the tumor cells. The most common clinical findings are pain, swelling in the preauricular region, and a reduced range of joint motion. Metastasis from a distant site may occur in the TMJ region, but the clinical signs and symptoms usually resemble those of common temporomandibular disorders and most often include unilateral facial swelling, a limitation of mandibular mobility, pain, and mandibular deviation. In patients who do not respond to treatment, the clinician should reconsider the initial diagnosis and include in the differential diagnosis the possibility of a malignant lesion. CBCT is very important in the diagnosis of malignancies. Malignant tumors are characterized by bone destruction with poorly defined borders and irregular margins, erosion of the cortical plates, and minimal expansion. Pathologic calcifications and condylar deformity may be detected. In case of suspected malignancy, CBCT examination should be followed up with other imaging modalities, such as MRI, CT, nuclear scan, or positron emission tomography.

Malignant neoplasms seen in the TMJs include primary malignancy or metastasis, chondrosarcoma, osteosarcoma, synovial sarcoma, and fibrosarcoma. Parotid salivary gland malignancies, rhabdomyosarcoma, and regional carcinomas may extend into the TMJ. Metastatic lesions are most common from the breast, kidney, lung, colon, prostate, and/or thyroid. Bone destruction presents as ill-defined and irregular in shape. Chondrosarcoma presents as discrete soft-tissue calcifications with destruction.

Differential Interpretation

Differential interpretation includes severe DJD but will have more peripheral bone destruction, osteophyte(s), and no soft-tissue swelling or mass. Sarcoma and other tumors have more central destruction of bone.

Treatment

Treatment includes wide surgical removal. For metastatic lesions, treatment options include palliative, radiation, and chemotherapy, if indicated.

References

Isberg, A. (2001). *Temporomandibular Joint Dysfunction, A Practitioner's Guide.* ISIS Medical Media.

Larheim, T. A., and Westesson, P. L. (2006). *Maxillofacial Imaging.* Springer.

Mallaya, S., and Lam, E. (Ed.). (2019). *White and Pharaoh's Oral Radiology: Principles and Interpretation.* Mosby.

Som, P. M., and Curtin, H. D. (2003). *Head and Neck Imaging,* Volume **1**. Mosby, pp. 995–1050.

11

Implants

Gayle Tieszen Reardon and Shawneen M. Gonzalez

Introduction

Diagnostic imaging helps develop and implement a cohesive and comprehensive treatment plan for the implant team and patient. The objectives of diagnostic imaging depend on the amount and type of information required and the time period of the treatment rendered. The decision of when to image along with which imaging modality to use depends on the integration of these factors and can be organized into three phases.

Phase One is the pre-prosthetic implant imaging phase and involves all past radiologic examinations as well as new radiologic examinations chosen to assist the implant team in determining the patient's final comprehensive treatment plan. The objectives of this phase of imaging include all necessary surgical and prosthetic information to determine the quantity, quality, and angulations of bone; the relationship of critical structures to the prospective implant sites; and the presence or absence of disease at the proposed surgery sites.

Phase Two is the surgical and interventional implant imaging phase and is focused on assisting in the surgical and prosthetic intervention of the patient. The objectives of this phase are to evaluate the surgery sites during and immediately after surgery, assist in the optimal position and orientation of dental implants, evaluate the healing and integration phase of implant surgery, and ensure that abutment position and prosthesis fabrication are appropriate.

Phase Three is the post-prosthetic implant imaging phase that commences just after the prosthesis placement and continues for the functional life of the dental implant(s). The objectives here are to evaluate the long-term maintenance of implant rigid fixation and function, including the crestal bone levels around each implant, and to evaluate the implant complex.

This chapter covers aspects regarding implant placement including accuracy of measurements, Hounsfield units, and mandibular nerve tracing. This chapter will not go into depth about stent construction or different software applications capable of these diagnostic criteria.

Interpretation Basics of Cone Beam Computed Tomography, Second Edition.
Edited by Shawneen M. Gonzalez.
© 2021 John Wiley & Sons, Inc. Published 2021 by John Wiley & Sons, Inc.
Companion website: www.wiley.com/go/gonzalez/interpretation

American Academy of Oral and Maxillofacial Radiology (AAOMR) Recommendations

In 2000, the AAOMR recommended some form of cross-sectional imaging for implant cases, further stating that conventional cross-sectional tomography was the "method of choice" for gaining the needed information. Since this original statement, cone beam computed tomography (CBCT) availability has increased. The AAOMR published a position statement on implants imaging specifically regarding CBCT use in June of 2012 with 11 primary recommendations.

Phase One Imaging: Initial Examination

Recommendation 1

Panoramic radiography should be used as the imaging modality of choice in the initial evaluation of the dental implant patient.

Pantomographs or panoramic radiograph units show information about both the maxilla and mandible and associated structures that may create issues with implant placement such as the mandibular nerve and maxillary sinuses. Accuracy of measurements on pantomographs is not reliable, with a relatively constant vertical magnification error of approximately 10% and a horizontal magnification error of approximately 20%, variables depending on the anatomical location, the patient positioning, the focus object distance, and the relative location of the rotation center for the x-ray system. Patient positioning is likely the most common factor contributing to the errors associated with panoramic radiography.

Recommendation 2

Use intraoral periapical radiography to supplement the preliminary information from panoramic radiography.

Periapical radiographs have a high spatial resolution showing minute detail. Again, as with pantomographs, error in positioning of the image receptor can create distortion and magnification errors in the final image, making accurate measurements impossible. The long cone paralleling technique eliminates distortion and limits magnification to less than 10%. In terms of Phase One pre-prosthetic implant imaging, the objectives include (1) A useful high-yield modality for ruling out local bone or dental disease; (2) of limited value in determining quantity because the image is magnified, may be distorted, and does not depict the third dimension of bone width; (3) of limited value in determining bone density or mineralization; and (4) of value in identifying critical structures but of little use in depicting the spatial relationship between the structures and the proposed implant site(s).

Recommendation 3

Do not use cross-sectional imaging, including CBCT, as an initial diagnostic imaging examination.

In 2000, the AAOMR stated, "After reviewing the current literature, they recommended some form of cross-sectional imaging be used for implant cases and that *conventional cross-sectional tomography be the method of choice for gaining this information for most patients receiving implant.*" Since then, the introduction and increased use of maxillofacial CBCT has had an impact on the availability of digital, cross-sectional imaging and expanded imaging clinical applications for dental implant imaging.

In 2012, it was noted that there had been a dramatic conceptual shift from a surgically driven to a prosthetically driven approach to dental implant therapy. It was no longer acceptable practice to place implants in alveolar bone without a previously developed plan for prosthetic restoration. Thus, it was considered important to optimize implant and avoid surgical complications for the clinician by having full knowledge of oral bone anatomy so that any osseous topography and bone volume excesses/deficiencies could be corrected prior to implant placement. It became accepted practice to dichotomize dental implant placement difficulty as either straightforward or complex based upon specific, patient presenting characteristics. A straightforward case was defined as a case where "the desired tooth position was clear" and where the surgical procedure involved minimal anatomical risk, with no need for significant hard- or soft-tissue grafting or modification of anatomical structures.

Conversely, a complex case was one for which the tooth position was "not easily identifiable" with a possible need for "extensive hard- and soft-tissue grafting" of the residual alveolar ridge.

Pre-operative Site-Specific Imaging

Pre-surgical assessment guidelines underscore the need for accurate assessment of bone volume and location of adjacent anatomical structures in relation to prosthetically derived, dental implant positioning.

Imaging for pre-surgical, dental implant planning must provide information supportive of the following goals:

1. *Establish the morphologic characteristics of residual alveolar ridge (RAR).* The RAR includes considerations of bone volume and quality. Vertical bone height, horizontal width, and edentulous saddle length determine the amount of bone volume available for implant fixture placement. This information is necessary to match the available bone dimensions of the implant(s). Moderate deficiencies in horizontal and vertical bone may be corrected by augmentation procedures at the time of the osteotomies and fixture placements. Severe deficiencies may require prior surgical procedures such as ridge augmentations. Excessive or irregular vertical alveolar bone may likewise require pre-prosthetic or simultaneous alveoloplasty.

   It is generally agreed that dental implant success depends on oral bone quality. Bone quality is considered "good" when there is enough cortical and trabecular bone to hold the implant securely, a requirement for osseointegration. Bone quality is considered poor when there is inadequate oral bone to hold the implant securely. Oral radiographic procedures are thought to be useful in assessing bone quality; however, there are few studies that have been devoted to assessing oral bone quality for implant placements. Better information is needed in this area to inform surgical techniques, implant selection, and loading protocols.

2. *Determine the orientation of the RAR.* Assessment of the orientation and residual topography of the alveolar basal bone complex is helpful to determine whether or not there are variations that could compromise the alignment of the implant fixture with the planned prosthetic restoration.

3. *Identify local anatomic or pathologic conditions restricting implant placement.* In the maxilla, these include the incisor region (nasopalatine fossa and canal, nasal fossa), the canine region (canine fossa, nasal fossa), and the premolar/molar region (floor of the maxillary sinus). In the mandible these include the incisor region (lingual foramen), canine/premolar region (mental foramen), and molar region (submandibular gland fossa and mandibular canal, which contains the neurovascular bundle).

4. *Match imaging findings with the prosthetic plan.* Radiographic images are not only used for prosthetic planning but also to construct surgical templates to guide the surgical procedures and implant placement. Surgical guides are increasing in use because of a number of clinical advantages including increased practitioner confidence and reduced operating time. Most studies indicate that panoramic and intraoral periapical data alone are inadequate to accomplish these goals and provide insufficient information to determine treatment difficulty.

Recommendation 4

The radiographic examination of any potential implant site should include cross-sectional imaging orthogonal to the site of interest.

This recommendation is consistent with the AAOMR's stance in 2000. Cross-sectional imaging techniques produce in-focus, thin-section images. Cross-sectional images can be produced with conventional tomography, panoramic-based scanography and tomography, CBCT, and computed tomography (CT). The main advantage of these images for implant dentistry is that they minimize or completely eliminate anatomic superimposition. Image sections perpendicular to the long axis of the region of interest are referred to as cross-sectional or trans-axial images. Cross-sectional images provide optimal accuracy for visualizing the bony architecture of the jaws. This allows for visualization of ridge morphology and bone quality in the area of the proposed implant(s) placement.

Recommendation 5

CBCT should be considered as the imaging modality of choice for pre-operative cross-sectional imaging of potential implant sites. The use of CBCT is lower radiation dose compared to traditional CT. The abbreviation CT represents scanners that use multi-row, detector arrays.

Data acquisition in CT has evolved over the past four decades with four generations of CT scanners. The most advanced systems use fan-beam radiation and multiple detector arrays. Usually, one source of fan-beam radiation is used. The user makes selections to define the spatial resolution, field of view, and image sharpness. As the object being scanned is translated through the CT scanner, the object attenuates the x-ray beam, and the attenuated x-ray beam data are collected by detector arrays. Mathematical formulas are used to reconstruct the volumetric and/or multi-planar images. The multi-planar reconstructions have various image thicknesses and may be in any image plane. The images are undistorted, calibrated for dimensional accuracy, and have high soft-tissue and hard-tissue contract resolution. CT is relatively expensive and is most commonly used in medical radiology departments and hospitals.

Recommendation 6

CBCT should be considered when clinical conditions indicate a need for augmentation procedures or site development before placement of dental implants. This includes areas of possible bone grafts including (1) maxillary sinus augmentation, (2) block or particulate bone grafting, (3) ramus or symphysis grafting, (4) assessment of impacted teeth in the field of interest, and (5) evaluation of prior traumatic injury.

Recommendation 7

CBCT imaging should be considered if bone reconstruction and augmentation procedures have been performed to treat bone volume deficiencies prior to implant placement. The CBCT will help assess the quality and integration of the bone graft, confirming that there is now adequate bone for implant placement.

Postoperative Imaging

Postoperative imaging after dental implant placement is used to confirm the location of the fixture at the implant insertion. From year 3 to year 5 and beyond, imaging is used to assess the bone–implant interface and marginal peri-implant bone height. Due to partial volume averaging, beam hardening, and streak artifacts that obscure subtle changes in marginal and peri-implant bone, intraoral radiography is superior to that of CBCT resolution for the detection of subtle bone changes.

Recommendation 8

In the absence of clinical signs or symptoms, use intraoral periapical radiography for the postoperative assessment of implants. Panoramic radiographs may be indicated for more extensive implant therapy cases.

Radiographs are used to assess the bone–implant interface and whether the implant shows adequate osseointegration over time. CBCT images are not recommended due to partial volume averaging, beam hardening, and streak artifacts created by the metal implant and thus obscuring the implant–bone interface.

Recommendation 9

Use cross-sectional imaging (CBCT) immediately postoperatively only if the patient presents with implant mobility or altered sensation, especially if the fixture is in the posterior mandible.

The immediate CBCT use is to evaluate whether there has been nerve involvement, especially in the posterior mandible.

Recommendation 10

Do not use CBCT imaging for periodic review of clinically asymptomatic implants. Implant failure, owing either to biological or mechanical causes, requires a complete assessment to characterize the existing defect, plan for surgical removal and corrective procedures, and identify the effect of surgery or the defect on adjacent structures.

Recommendation 11

Cross-sectional imaging, optimally CBCT, should be considered if implant retrieval is anticipated.

CBCT Image Development

CT images are the result of data collected by numerous detectors and ionizing chambers in the CT unit. The data collected by the detectors correspond to a composite of the absorption characteristics of the tissues and structures imaged. This information is transformed into images (raw data), which is reformatted into a voxel (digital) volume for evaluation and analysis.

The integration of digital imaging systems in the field of implant dentistry has significantly increased clinicians' diagnostic capabilities. A digital 2D image is described by an image matrix that has individual picture elements called pixels. A digital image is described by its width and height and pixels (i.e., 512 x 512). Each picture element, or pixel, has a discrete digital value that describes the image intensity at that particular point. The value of a pixel element is described by a scale, which may be as low as 8 bits (256 values) or as high as 12 bits (4096 values) for black and white imaging systems or 36 bits (65 billion values) for color imaging systems.

A digital 3D image is described not only by its width and height of pixels but also by its depth and thickness. An imaging volume or 3D characterization of the patient is produced by contiguous images that produce a 3D structure of volume elements. Each volume element has a value that describes its intensity level. Typically, 3D modalities have an intensity scale of 12 bits or 4096 values. The 2D digital images are composed of pixels (2D) and voxels (3D) picture elements. Pixels and voxels possess attributes of size, location, and gray-scale value. Each voxel and pixel displayed is characterized by a numerical value that represents the density of the tissues. This is termed the CT number.

A specific shade of gray or density value is assigned to each CT number that comprises the images.

CT images are inherently 3D images that are typically 512 x 512 pixels with a thickness described by the slice spacing of the imaging technique. Each voxel has a value, referred to in Hounsfield units, that describes the density of each image. The range of these units is -1000 (air) to +3000 (enamel) Hounsfield units. Most CT scanners are standardized with a Hounsfield value of 0 for water. The CT density scale is quantitative and meaningful in identifying and differentiating structures and tissues.

Gray Values and Hounsfield Units

A Hounsfield unit (HU) is "the numeric information contained in each pixel of a CT image. It is related to the composition and nature of the tissue imaged and is used to represent the density of tissue" (Medical Dictionary). As just mentioned, Hounsfield units have a wide range from –1000 to +3000 (Table 11.1). Bone will present with a HU of +400 and increase as it becomes denser, such as in the case of cortical bone. CBCT imaging is primarily a hard-tissue imaging modality, whereas traditional medical CT imaging can accurately image both hard-tissue and soft-tissue densities. Varying gray levels are still seen on scans of soft tissues of different densities. Hounsfield units used in CBCT imaging are actually gray values used with linear attenuation coefficients (Figure 11.1). Studies have shown strong correlation between gray levels and Hounsfield units. Hounsfield unit accuracy varies and represents differences attributable to patient positioning, patient size, and imaging artifacts. When used for implant placement, the Hounsfield units should be considered an idea of bone density rather than an exact unit of bone density.

Table 11.1. Hounsfield units for various tissues frequently captured on a CBCT scan.

Material	Hounsfield units
Air	1000
Water	0
Muscle	35–70
Fibrous tissue	60–90
Cartilage	80–130
Trabecular bone	150–900
Cortical bone	900–1800
Dentin	1600–2400
Enamel	2500–3000

(a)   (b)

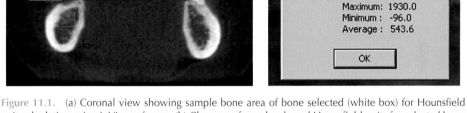

Figure 11.1.   (a) Coronal view showing sample bone area of bone selected (white box) for Hounsfield unit calculation using InVivo software. (b) Close-up of gray levels and Hounsfield units for selected bone using InVivo software. Source: Anatomage Inc.

Bone Density: A Key Determinant for Treatment Planning

The treatment plan should first consider the final prosthesis options and determine the prosthesis type indicated for the specific patient in question. The key implant positions for the prosthesis may then be determined using a biomechanical perspective. The additional number of implants required to support the specific restoration may then be established related to the amount of force generated by the patient because stress equals force divided by area. The next consideration to determine the additional implant number and size to support the restoration is the bone density in the sites of the implant abutments.

The external (cortical) and internal (trabecular) structure of bone may be described by the terms "quality" or "density," which reflects a number of biomechanical properties, such as strength, modulus of elasticity, bone–implant contact percent, and stress distribution around a loaded endosteal implant. It is the external and internal architecture of bone that controls virtually every facet of the practice of implant dentistry. Bone density is the determining factor in dental implant treatment planning, the surgical approach, the implant design, the healing time, and the need for initial progressive bone loading during prosthetic reconstruction.

The densest bone is typically observed in the anterior mandible, followed by the anterior maxilla and posterior mandible, and the least dense bone is usually found in the posterior maxilla. When considering implant survival, researchers have reported an approximate 10% greater success rate in the anterior mandible as compared with the anterior maxilla.

In addition to arch location, reported failure rates have also been related to the quality of bone. Reduced implant survival most often is more related to bone density than to arch location. Over the years, many independent clinical groups, following standardized surgical and prosthetic protocols, documented the indisputable influence of bone density on clinical success, concluding that bone density is considered a key determinant for clinical success for any potential implant site. The strength of the bone is directly related to the bone density (Table 11.2).

In situations where the bone types are softer, the treatment plan may be altered to compensate for the softer bone. In other words, after the prosthetic option, key implant position(s), and patient force factors have been determined, the bone density in the implant sites should be evaluated to modify the treatment plan where needed. The treatment plan can be modified by reducing the force on the prosthesis or increasing the area of load by increasing the number of implants placed, or by changing the size, design, and/or surface of the dental implants used. Typically, increasing the number of implants used is the most effective method of decreasing the stress upon the implant system for all bone densities.

Linear Measurement Accuracy

The accuracy of linear and volumetric measurements with CBCT is very important prior to implant placement to ensure preventing damage to adjacent vital structures such as the mandibular nerve canal and/or maxillary sinuses. Linear measurements using dry skulls without soft tissue and with soft tissue were shown to have no statistical difference in measurements made on both the skulls and CBCT scan (Figure 11.2). Varying voxel size from 0.2 mm to 0.4 mm showed no statistical

Table 11.2. Hounsfield units for various bone densities as captured on a CBCT scan.

Bone quality	Hounsfield units
D1	1250
D2	850–1250
D3	350–850
D4	150–350
D5	<150

(a)

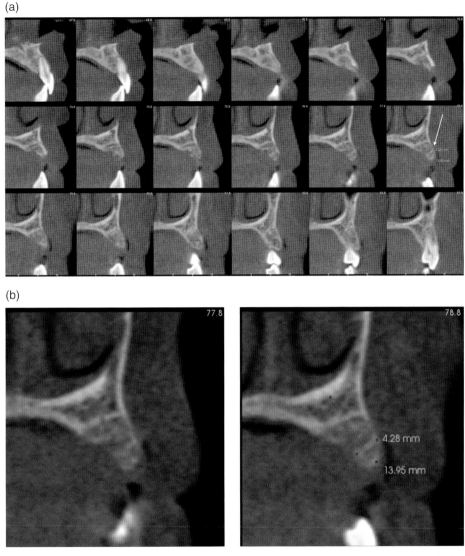

(b)

Figure 11.2.   (a) Cross-sectional slices through anterior maxilla with 1.0 mm spacing between each slice and sample measurements (white arrow). (b) Close-up of cross-sectional slices with measurements.

difference in linear measurements of width and height of dry skulls. This allows a practitioner to use a larger voxel size for implant placement, creating a reduction in radiation exposure to the patient.

Mandibular Canal

The location of the mandibular canal and anterior extension of the mandibular canal (sometimes referred to as mandibular incisive canal) are important when placing implants in the mandible. On pantomographs, the anterior extension of the mandibular canal is visible in up to approximately 51.7% of patients. On CBCT scans, the mandibular canal is clearly visible on approximately 53% to 87.9% of patients (Figures 11.3–11.5). When identifying the mandibular canal, cross-sectional slices, axial views, and sagittal views (Figure 11.6) are commonly used. Acquiring a CBCT does not guarantee that a difficult to view mandibular canal will be evident.

Virtual Implant Placement Software

There are several different software options regarding virtual implant placement. Due to the wide scope of different programs, this chapter will merely show examples of what those virtual implants look like in the CBCT software and cross-sectional views (Figure 11.7). For more information on specific software options, it is recommended to contact the company directly.

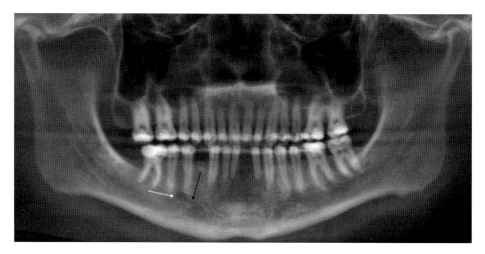

Figure 11.3. Reconstructed pantomograph from a CBCT scan showing the anterior extension of the right mandibular canal (black arrow) inferiorly and anteriorly from the mental foramen (white arrow) as a thin radiolucent line.

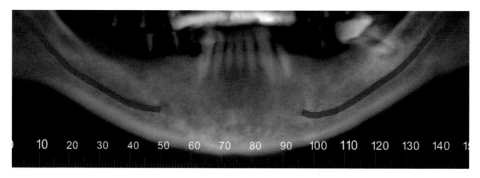

Figure 11.4. Reconstructed pantomograph from a CBCT scan showing right and left mandibular canal noted as red bands.

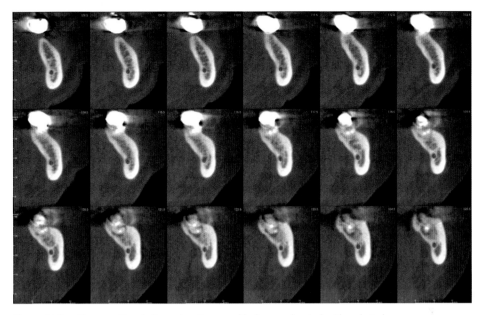

Figure 11.5. Cross-sectional views showing mandibular canal noted with red circles.

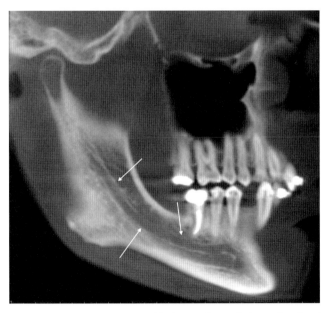

Figure 11.6. Rotated sagittal view showing mandibular canal as radiolucent band with thin radiopaque borders (white arrows).

(a)

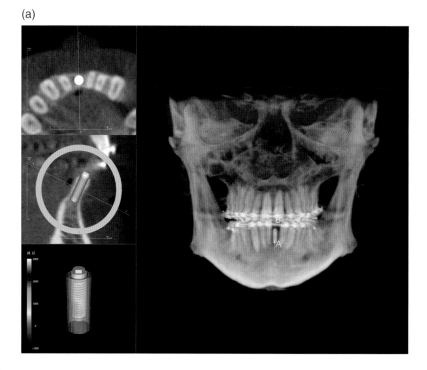

(b)

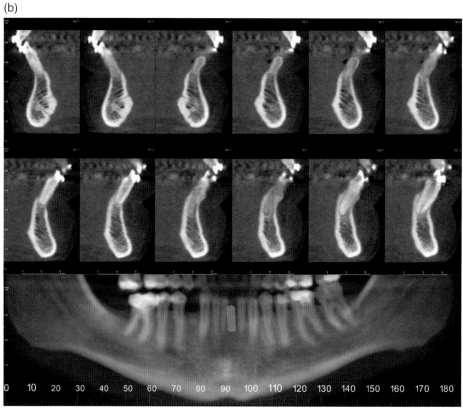

Figure 11.7.   (a) Implant screen using InVivo software with corresponding axial (top left box) and single cross-sectional slice (middle left box) and Hounsfield units (bottom left box). (b) Cross-sectional slices with 1.0 mm spacing showing virtual implant (green) and surrounding bone.

References

Ganguly, R., Ruprecht, A., Vincent, S., et al. (2011). Accuracy of linear measurement in the Galileos cone beam computed tomography under simulated clinical conditions. *Dentomaxillofac Radiol*, **40**, 299–305.

Jalili, M. R., Esmaeelinejad, M., Bayat, M., et al. (2012). Appearance of anatomical structures of mandible on panoramic radiographs in Iranian population. *Acta Odontol Scand*, **70**, 384–9.

Klinge, B., Petersson, A., Maly, P. (1989). Location of the mandibular canal: comparison of macroscopic findings, conventional radiography, and computed tomography. *Int J Oral Maxillofac Implants*, **4**, 327–32.

Lofthag-Hansen, S., Grondahl, K., Ekestubbe, A. (2009). Cone-beam CT for preoperative implant planning in the posterior mandible: visibility of anatomic landmarks. *Clin Implant Dent Relat Res*, **11**, 246–55.

Mah, P., Reeves, T. E., McDavid, W. D. (2010). Deriving Hounsfield units using grey levels in cone beam computed tomography. *Dentomaxillofac Radiol*, **39**, 323–25. Medical Dictionary. (http://medical-dictionary.thefreedictionary.com/Hounsfield+unit).

Oliveira-Santos, C., Capelozza, A. L. A., Dezzoti, M. S. G., et al. Visibility of the mandibular canal on CBCT cross-sectional images. *J Appl Oral Sci*, **19**, 240–3.

Parsa, A., Ibrahim, N., Hassan, B., et al. (2012). Reliability of voxel gray values in cone beam computed tomography for preoperative implant planning assessment. *Int J Oral Maxillofac Implants*, **27**, 1438–42.

Ping, H. S., and Kandaiya, S. (2012). The influence of the patient size and geometry on cone beam-computed tomography Hounsfield unit. *J Med Phys*, **37**, 155–8.

Reeves, T. E., Mah, P., McDavid, W. D. (2012). Deriving Hounsfield units using grey levels in cone beam CT: a clinical application. *Dentomaxillofac Radiol*, **41**, 500–8.

Sheikhi, M., Ghorbanizadeh, S., Abdinian, M., et al. (2012). Accuracy of linear measurements of Galileos cone beam computed tomography in normal and different head positions. *Int J Dent*, **2012**, 214954.

Torres, M. G. G., Campos, P. S. F., Segundo, N. P. N., et al. (2012). Accuracy of linear measurements in cone beam computed tomography with different voxel sizes. *Implant Dent*, **21**, 150–5.

Tyndall, D. A., Price, J. P., Tetradis, S., et al. (2012). Position statement of the American Academy of Oral and Maxillofacial Radiology on selection criteria for the use of radiology in dental implantology with emphasis on cone beam computed tomography. *Oral Surg Oral Med Oral Pathol Oral Radiol*, **113**, 817–26.

Zoller, J. E., and Nuegebauer, J. (2008). *Cone-beam Volumetric Imaging in Dental, Oral and Maxillofacial Medicine*. Quintessence, Germany.

Appendix   Sample Reports

Shawneen M. Gonzalez

Introduction

This appendix includes sample reports of different areas captured on cone beam computed tomography (CBCT) scans. The three reports show example reports for CBCT scans made for various reasons. The general health report is an example of a report for a CBCT scan received with no specific area of interest to review. The pathology report is an example of a report for a CBCT scan where there was obvious pathosis and the practitioner wanted more information about the nature and location of the disease process prior to determining the next treatment step. The endodontic report is an example of a report for a CBCT scan made due to endodontic issues.

Interpretation Basics of Cone Beam Computed Tomography, Second Edition.
Edited by Shawneen M. Gonzalez.
© 2021 John Wiley & Sons, Inc. Published 2021 by John Wiley & Sons, Inc.
Companion website: www.wiley.com/go/gonzalez/interpretation

General Health Report

Oral Radiology Reports

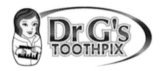

Shawneen M Gonzalez, DDS, MS
Diplomate ABOMR

Referring Dr.
Patient:

Indication: General pathology review.
Pertinent History: None given.
Protocol: A cone beam CT dataset (Carestream CS 8100, 90kVp, 5mA, 15s, 0.07mm) of the mandible was acquired and reconstructed on xx xx, xxxx. The resultant axial, coronal, sagittal, panoramic and orthoradial reconstructions were examined.
Image Quality: Streaking / Beam hardening.

Teeth / Jaws:

i = implant, rf = root fragment, p = pontic, S = supernumerary tooth, *=portions of tooth visualized

			*	*	*	*	*	*	*
26*	25		24	23	22	21	20	p	18*

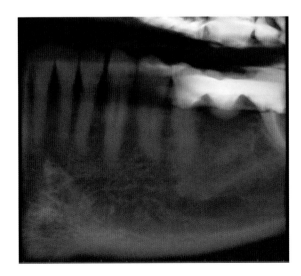

Patient Name: Report Number:

Shawneen M Gonzalez, DDS, MS
Diplomate ABOMR

There are two mental foramina of the left side of the mandible (variant of normal anatomy).

Rotated sagittal and 3D reconstruction views

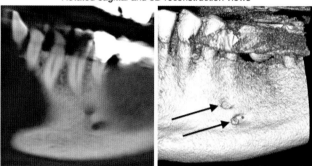

Two mental foramina (black arrows)

There are no periapical inflammatory lesions detected. There are no abnormalities detected within the bone trabeculation.

Soft Tissues:
No abnormalities detected.

Interpretation

1. Two mental foramina = left side of mandible.
2. No periapical inflammatory lesions detected.

This is a consultative report only and is not intended to be a definitive diagnosis or treatment plan.

Shawneen M Gonzalez, DDS, MS
Diplomate, American Board of Oral and Maxillofacial Radiology

Patient Name: Report Number:

Pathology Report

Oral Radiology Reports

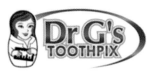

Shawneen M Gonzalez, DDS, MS
Diplomate ABOMR

Referring Dr.
Patient:

Indication: Evaluation of resorption.
Pertinent History: None given.
Protocol: A cone beam CT dataset (Carestream CS 9300, 90kVp, 4mA, 8s, 0.18mm) of the maxilla and mandible was acquired and reconstructed on xx xx, xxxx. The resultant axial, coronal, sagittal, panoramic and orthoradial reconstructions were examined.
Image Quality: Streaking / Beam hardening.

Teeth / Jaws:

i = implant, rf = root fragment, p = pontic, S = supernumerary tooth, *=portions of tooth visualized

2	3	4	5	6	7	8	9	10	11	12	13	14	15
31	30	29	28	27	26	25	24	23	22	21	20	19	18

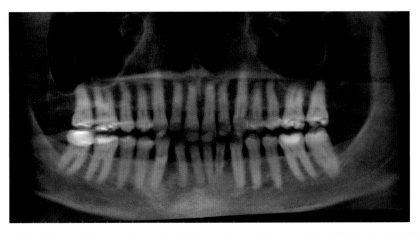

There is invasive cervical resorption on the facial root surface of the mandibular left lateral incisor (#23). The resorption appears stable from xx xxxx scan. *Additional images at end of report*

Oral Radiology Reports

Shawneen M Gonzalez, DDS, MS
Diplomate ABOMR

Rotated axial and sagittal views

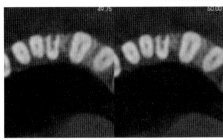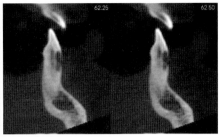

External resorption # 23

There is internal resorption of the mandibular right canine (#27) inferior to the existing facial restoration. The resorption appears stable from xx xxxx scan.

Coronal and sagittal views

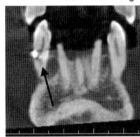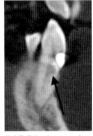

Suggestive internal resorption # 27 (black arrow)

There is suggestive focal idiopathic osteosclerosis (cortical bone hyperplasia - variant of normal bone trabeculation) apical to the mandibular left canine (#22).

Patient Name: Report Number:

There is a well-defined, round, radiolucent area between the roots of the mandibular right lateral incisor (#26) and canine (#22). There is thinning of the facial cortical plate. A differential interpretation includes lateral periodontal cyst, odontogenic keratocyst and lateral rarefying osteitis (abscess, cyst and/or granuloma). The radiolucent area appears stable from xx xxxx scan.

Axial and coronal views

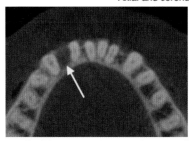 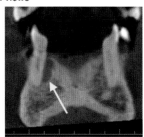

Radiolucent area between the roots of # 26 and # 27 (yellow arrow)

There is a well-defined, round, radiolucent area between the roots of the maxillary left lateral incisor (#10) and canine (#11). A differential interpretation includes a lateral periodontal cyst and odontogenic keratocyst.

Axial and coronal views

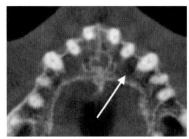 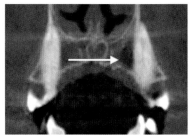

Radiolucent area between roots of # 10 and # 11 (white arrow)

There are no periapical inflammatory lesions detected.

Paranasal Sinuses:
The visualized borders of the paranasal sinuses appear to be intact. There is a radiopaque, dome-shaped mass in the left maxillary sinus. The appearance is consistent with a mucous retention pseudocyst. The bilateral ostiomeatal units are patent.

Nasal Cavity:
There is bilateral paradoxical curvature (reverse curvature - developmental variant of normal anatomy) associated with the middle conchae. The nasal septum is deviated.

Shawneen M Gonzalez, DDS, MS
Diplomate ABOMR

Airway:
No abnormalities detected.

Skull:
No abnormalities detected.

Soft Tissues:
No abnormalities detected.

Interpretation

1. Invasive cervical resorption = # 23. Stable from xx xxxx scan.
2. Internal resorption = # 27. Stable from xx xxxx scan.
3. Well-defined, round radiolucent area between the roots of # 26 and # 27. Differential interpretation includes lateral periodontal cyst, odontogenic keratocyst and lateral rarefying osteitis (abscess, cyst and/or granuloma). Stable from xx xxxx scan.
4. Well-defined, round radiolucent area between the roots of # 10 and # 11. Differential interpretation includes lateral periodontal cyst and odontogenic keratocyst.
5. No periapical inflammatory lesions detected.

This is a consultative report only and is not intended to be a definitive diagnosis or treatment plan.

Shawneen M Gonzalez, DDS, MS
Diplomate, American Board of Oral and Maxillofacial Radiology

Patient Name: Report Number:

Oral Radiology Reports

Shawneen M Gonzalez, DDS, MS
Diplomate ABOMR

Rotated axial views = # 23

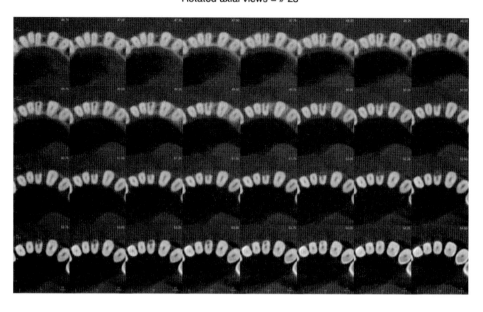

Rotated sagittal views # 23

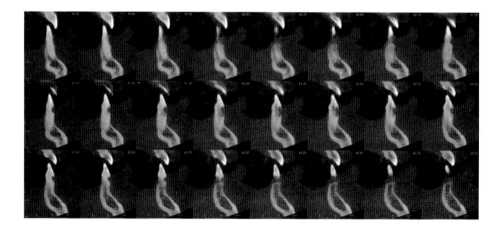

Patient Name: **Report Number:**

Endodontic Report

Oral Radiology Reports

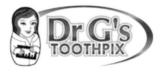

Shawneen M Gonzalez, DDS, MS
Diplomate ABOMR

Referring Dr.
Patient:

Indication: Evaluate # 14.
Pertinent History: None given.
Protocol: A cone beam CT dataset (Carestream CS 9000, 68kVp, 6mA, 10.8s, 0.08mm) of the maxilla was acquired and reconstructed on xx xx, xxxx. The resultant axial, coronal, sagittal, panoramic and orthoradial reconstructions were examined.
Image Quality: Streaking / Beam hardening.

Teeth / Jaws:

i = implant, rf = root fragment, p = pontic, S = supernumerary tooth, *=portions of tooth visualized

	9*	10*	11	12	13	14	15
							*

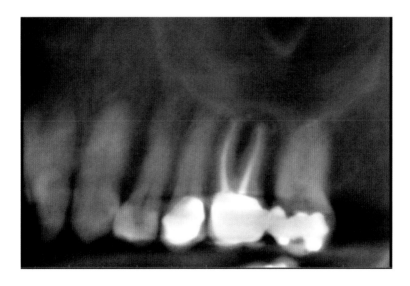

There are multiple well-defined, radiolucent areas at the apices of the endodontically treated maxillary left first molar (#14). There are discontinuities of the palatal and buccal cortical plates. There is a suggestive discontinuity of the floor of the left maxillary sinus. The appearance is suggestive of rarefying osteitis (abscess, cyst and/or granuloma). *Additional images at end of report*

Rotated coronal and sagittal views

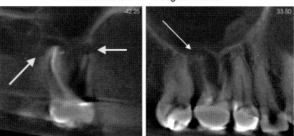

Discontinuities of buccal and palatal cortical plates # 14 (yellow arrows)
Suggestive discontinuity of floor of the left maxillary sinus (white arrow)

There is internal resorption of the maxillary left second molar (#15) palatal root.

Axial, coronal and sagittal views

Internal resorption # 15 palatal root (black arrow)

Patient Name: Report Number:

Shawneen M Gonzalez, DDS, MS
Diplomate ABOMR

Paranasal Sinuses:
There is a suggestive discontinuity of the floor of the left maxillary sinus at the first molar (#14) area.
There is soft tissue thickening of the left maxillary sinus, consistent with sinusitis.

Nasal Cavity:
No abnormalities detected.

Soft Tissues:
No abnormalities detected.

Interpretation

1. Suggestive rarefying osteitis = # 14.
2. Discontinuities of buccal and palatal cortical plates = # 14 area.
3. Suggestive discontinuity of the floor of the left maxillary sinus = # 14 area.
4. Sinusitis = left maxillary sinus.
5. Internal resorption = # 15 palatal root.

This is a consultative report only and is not intended to be a definitive diagnosis or treatment plan.

Shawneen M Gonzalez, DDS, MS
Diplomate, American Board of Oral and Maxillofacial Radiology

Patient Name: Report Number:

Oral Radiology Reports

Shawneen M Gonzalez, DDS, MS
Diplomate ABOMR

Rotated coronal views = # 14

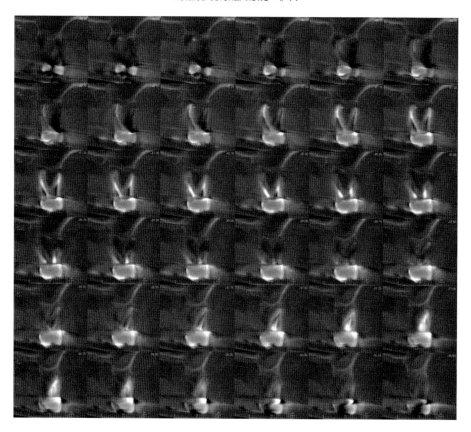

Patient Name: **Report Number:**

Shawneen M Gonzalez, DDS, MS
Diplomate ABOMR

Oral Radiology Reports

Rotated sagittal views = # 14

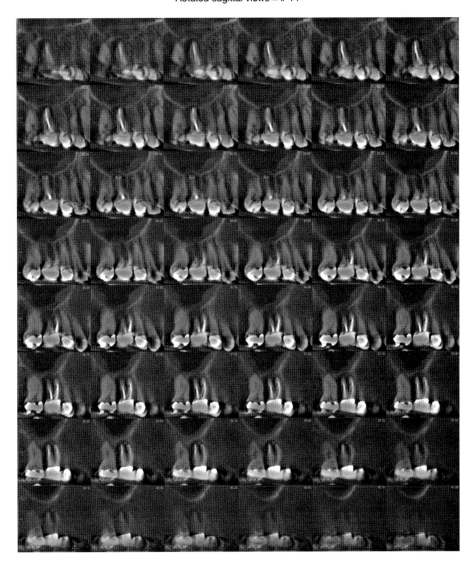

Patient Name: Report Number:

Index

Interpretation Basics of Cone Beam Computed Tomography, Second Edition.
Edited by Shawneen M. Gonzalez.
© 2021 John Wiley & Sons, Inc. Published 2021 by John Wiley & Sons, Inc.
Companion website: www.wiley.com/go/gonzalez/interpretation